Nursing Research Using Participatory Action Research

Mary de Chesnay, PhD, RN, PMHCNS-BC, FAAN, is professor at Kennesaw State University, School of Nursing, Kennesaw, Georgia. She has received 13 research grants and has authored two books: *Sex Trafficking: A Clinical Guide for Nurses* (Springer Publishing) and the AJN Book of the Year Award winner, *Caring for the Vulnerable: Perspectives in Nursing Theory, Practice and Research*, now in its third edition (with a fourth edition to be published in 2015). Dr. de Chesnay has published over 21 journal articles in *Qualitative Health Research, Journal of Nursing Management, International Journal of Medicine & Law*, and others. A former dean and endowed chair, she reviews for a variety of professional journals. Dr. de Chesnay is a noted expert on qualitative research and a founding member and first vice president of the Southern Nursing Research Society.

Nursing Research Using Participatory Action Research

Qualitative Designs and Methods in Nursing

Mary de Chesnay, PhD, RN, PMHCNS-BC, FAAN

Editor

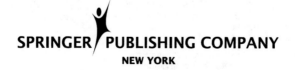

SPRINGER PUBLISHING COMPANY

NEW YORK

Springer Publishing Company, LLC
11 West 42nd Street
New York, NY 10036
www.springerpub.com

Acquisitions Editor: Joseph Morita
Production Editor: Kris Parrish
Composition: Exeter Premedia Services Private Ltd.

ISBN: 978-0-8261-2613-9
e-book ISBN: 978-0-8261-2614-6

Set ISBN: 978-0-8261-7134-4
Set e-book ISBN: 978-0-8261-3015-0

14 15 16 17 / 5 4 3 2 1

The author and the publisher of this Work have made every effort to use sources believed to be reliable to provide information that is accurate and compatible with the standards generally accepted at the time of publication. Because medical science is continually advancing, our knowledge base continues to expand. Therefore, as new information becomes available, changes in procedures become necessary. We recommend that the reader always consult current research and specific institutional policies before performing any clinical procedure. The author and publisher shall not be liable for any special, consequential, or exemplary damages resulting, in whole or in part, from the readers' use of, or reliance on, the information contained in this book. The publisher has no responsibility for the persistence or accuracy of URLs for external or third-party Internet websites referred to in this publication and does not guarantee that any content on such websites is, or will remain, accurate or appropriate.

Library of Congress Cataloging-in-Publication Data
Nursing research using participatory action research : qualitative designs and methods in nursing / [edited by] Mary de Chesnay.
     p. ; cm.
  Includes bibliographical references and index.
  ISBN 978-0-8261-2613-9—ISBN 978-0-8261-2614-6 (e-book)
  I. de Chesnay, Mary, editor.
  [DNLM: 1. Nursing Research—methods. 2. Community-Based Participatory Research—methods. 3. Consumer Participation—methods. 4. Qualitative Research. 5. Research Design. WY 20.5]
  RT81.5
  610.73072—dc23
                                                                                          2014030146

Printed in the United States of America by Gasch Printing.

QUALITATIVE DESIGNS AND METHODS IN NURSING

Mary de Chesnay, PhD, RN, PMHCNS-BC, FAAN, Series Editor

Nursing Research Using Ethnography: Qualitative Designs and Methods in Nursing

Nursing Research Using Grounded Theory: Qualitative Designs and Methods in Nursing

Nursing Research Using Life History: Qualitative Designs and Methods in Nursing

Nursing Research Using Phenomenology: Qualitative Designs and Methods in Nursing

Nursing Research Using Historical Methods: Qualitative Designs and Methods in Nursing

Nursing Research Using Participatory Action Research: Qualitative Designs and Methods in Nursing

Nursing Research Using Data Analysis: Qualitative Designs and Methods in Nursing

For Dr. Joanne White and her husband, Dr. Richard White, whose efforts in Nicaragua exemplify the spirit of participatory action research and who inspired others to conduct these kinds of studies.

—MdC

CONTENTS

Contributors

Anne Watson Bongiorno, RN, PhD, APHN-BC, CNE, is associate professor of nursing at SUNY Plattsburgh, New York. Her work in nursing education includes positions as past chairperson of the Council on Nursing Education and membership of the Council of Ethics with the New York State Nurses Association. She serves as a nurse ethicist on several boards of ethics in her region and has taught ethics in both undergraduate and graduate programs. She has recently concluded a study of academic misconduct (in press) and is in the analysis phase of a qualitative study examining nursing and technology. She is particularly interested in the relationship between diversity and health disparity and in bringing awareness to students of the influence of their own worldview. Currently, she is working in the field with indigenous projects locally and abroad.

Joan L. Bottorff, PhD, RN, FCAHS, FAAN, is professor of nursing at the University of British Columbia, Okanagan campus, faculty of Health and Social Development. She is the director of the Institute for Healthy Living and Chronic Disease Prevention at the University of British Columbia.

Bonnie H. Bowie, PhD, MBA, RN, is associate professor and chair of the Psychosocial and Community Health Nursing Department at Seattle University College of Nursing. She has conducted community-based research and participatory action research on vulnerable populations throughout the Seattle area.

Karen Lucas Breda, PhD, RN, is associate professor of nursing at the University of Hartford in West Hartford, Connecticut, and president of the Council on Nursing and Anthropology (CONAA) of the Society for Applied Anthropology (SFAA). She has conducted participatory action research and explored issues of nursing professionalism and autonomy with practicing nurses. She is the director of Project Horizon, a network of community-driven advocacy partnerships among the University of Hartford and agencies serving urban community populations. She has conducted case study and ethnographic research and has written on globalization and the role of nursing in the modern era.

Lauren Clark, PhD, RN, FAAN, is professor of nursing at the University of Utah and chair of the Division of Health Systems and Community-Based Care. She is a past president of the Council on Nursing and Anthropology (CONAA) with a long-standing interest in culture, health, and health disparities. She has taught qualitative research and conducted ethnographic research on a variety of health topics. Most recently, she has studied early child feeding practices and obesity in Mexican immigrants and Mexican families and is currently working with an interdisciplinary team on disability and obesity prevention.

Mary de Chesnay, PhD, RN, PMHCNS-BC, FAAN, is professor of nursing at Kennesaw State University and secretary of the Council on Nursing and Anthropology (CONAA) of the Society for Applied Anthropology (SFAA). She has conducted ethnographic fieldwork and participatory action research in Latin America and the Caribbean. She has taught qualitative research at all levels in the United States and abroad in the roles of faculty, head of a department of research, dean, and endowed chair.

Jennifer Foster, PhD, MPH, CNM, FACNM, is clinical associate professor of nursing and associate in anthropology at Emory University. She is an at-large board member of the Council of Nursing and Anthropology (CONAA) of the Society for Applied Anthropology (SFAA), as well as a member of the Council of the Anthropology of Reproduction of the American Anthropological Association. Dr. Foster is a life member and fellow of the American College of Nurse-Midwives. She has conducted ethnographic fieldwork and participatory action research in Massachusetts, Georgia, and the Dominican Republic. She teaches qualitative methods in the doctoral program at Emory University and has conducted workshops in participatory research methods in Paraguay and Colombia.

Janet Katz, PhD, RN, is associate professor at the Washington State University College of Nursing. She works in nursing education and research to recruit and retain underserved populations into college and nursing. Dr. Katz has community expertise working with American Indian and Hispanic communities and youth, and research expertise in community-based participatory research. She is a coprincipal investigator of a community-based participatory research grant, "Substance Abuse and Mental Health Collaborative for

Rural American Indian Adolescents," from the National Institute of Minority Health Disparities (NIMHD) and principal investigator for "Nursing Pathways" funded by a Health Resources Services Administration Work Force Diversity grant. Dr. Katz also collaborates with a multidisciplinary team on an NIMHD grant, "Collaborative Action Towards Community Health," to improve health in native communities.

Patricia J. Kelly, PhD, MPH, APRN, is professor at the University of Missouri–Kansas City School of Nursing and Health Studies, associate dean for research, and coordinator of the PhD program. She has used a variety of methods in conducting research in community settings. Dr. Kelly teaches quantitative methods and community-based health interventions for graduate students.

Lorna Kendrick, PhD, PMHCNS-BC, is professor and UOPX Center for Health Engineering Research Fellow at the University of Phoenix, and member and past chair of the nominating committee of the Council on Nursing and Anthropology (CONAA) of the Society for Applied Anthropology (SFAA). She has conducted ethnographic fieldwork and participatory action research with young African American men on their perceptions of depression, as well as in Cuba, Alaska, Turkey, Argentina, Nigeria, and South Africa. She has also focused her research on untreated depression as a primary risk factor for early onset cardiovascular disease. She teaches qualitative and quantitative research courses at all levels in the United States and has taught an advanced nursing role course in Cape Town, South Africa.

Lauren Valk Lawson, DNP, RN, is a community health instructor with a focus on cross-cultural health at Seattle University College of Nursing. She is a recipient of a Nursing Faculty Initiative Grant and works with graduate students to complete an assessment and implementation of services to a homeless population.

Nicole Mareno, PhD, RN, is assistant professor of nursing at Kennesaw State University in Kennesaw, Georgia. Dr. Mareno has been studying childhood obesity and family weight management since 2006. Dr. Mareno's current research interests include childhood obesity prevention and treatment and cultural competence. She has conducted community-based participatory research and has experience using the photovoice data collection method.

Tommie Nelms, PhD, RN, is professor of nursing at Kennesaw State University. She is director of the WellStar School of Nursing and coordinator of the Doctor of Nursing Science program. She has a long history of conducting and directing phenomenological research and has been a student of Heideggerian philosophy and research for many years. Her research is mainly focused on practices of mothering, caring, and family.

Matthew Peters, RN, MSN, PhDc, works for Intermountain Healthcare in Salt Lake City, Utah, as a program manager for surgical services. At Intermountain, he is responsible for supporting groups of physicians and nurses in delivering the highest quality of care for patients at the lowest appropriate cost. He received a master's degree in nursing informatics from the College of Nursing at the University of Utah and is currently a PhD candidate. His research interest is in influencing clinician behavior using performance feedback created based on patient care data from electronic medical records.

Marie Truglio-Londrigan, PhD, RN, is professor at Pace University, College of Health Professions, Lienhard School of Nursing. She has conducted qualitative studies and participatory action research involving older adults. Dr. Truglio-Londrigan holds a baccalaureate degree from Herbert H. Lehman College, an MSN in Primary Health Care Nursing of the Aged from Seton Hall University, and a PhD in nursing from Adelphi University. Dr. Truglio-Londrigan has been a nurse since 1976 and has primarily practiced in public health, community, and long-term care. Most recently, she has held a faculty practice at Aging in America, the parent company for Morningside House in the Bronx, and prior to that, she served as a consultant for population-based practice at the Bergen County Department of Health Services in New Jersey. Her practice has focused primarily in the area of public and community health with a specialization in the care of older adults. She is a fellow of the New York Academy of Medicine and has participated in several evidence-based practice initiatives with DNP students. Her own research interests include shared decision making, health promotion, and disease prevention with an emphasis on patient-centered care.

Foreword

Nursing is a doing profession. We want to make life better for our patients, their families, and the communities in which they live. We do interventions. Participatory action research (PAR) provides us with two important principles for these interventions.

The first of these principles is *participation* and the importance of partnering with those being researched. Participants know their lives and their issues, and including—no, partnering with—these participants makes for extremely relevant research results. Just as we do patient-centered care, as nurses our focus should be on participant-centered research. We do not collect data and run. We give back to our participants and ensure that they have gained something from their interactions with researchers beyond the $10 gift card we are able to provide. While we as researchers have been privileged with the education that enables us to conduct research, participants have lived what we are investigating and studying. The exchange of expertise that happens in PAR projects ensures that we all benefit.

The second principle is *action*, with social change as a critical part of the outcome process of PAR. Action can focus on health issues (most common for nurses), around community issues such as environmental pollution, or around political and economic issues. Sustainability is an important part of action, since change occurs slowly. Can the curriculum or program that was implemented by the community group continue? Can participants use the information that they learned to secure legislative action? Can changes in healthy behaviors for individuals or communities endure? PAR outcomes move beyond the generation and dissemination of knowledge through manuscripts to include presentations and articles in venues accessible to members of the "researched" group, whether they are cancer survivors, incarcerated women, or whole communities linked by geography, demographics, or common interests.

Implementation of a PAR project is highly stimulating and demanding. Make no mistake: PAR is not necessarily an easy endeavor for a nurse researcher. But the results bring satisfaction on a professional, personal, and group or community level. One of the exciting things about PAR is its flexibility—qualitative, quantitative, mixed methods, ethnography, and needs assessments are all easily incorporated and welcomed. Your intellectual acumen will be put to the test as you consider which methods will be best suited for the goals of your project and how your community can be effectively trained. Attention must be simultaneously paid to both process and outcomes. But, as nurse researchers, we live in two worlds—that of our patients/clients/participants and that of academia. It is indeed a privilege to be able to move back and forth between both of these worlds.

Challenges do exist. Institutional review boards may not appreciate the fact that we want all participants to also serve as data collectors and be part of the analysis process. Getting everyone certified in the basics of the protection of human subjects can be unwieldy, but it is possible. Figuring out how to train members of the researched group to give presentations, to be the voice for local publicity about a project, and to include them in manuscript writing takes time and dedication to the task. It is also extremely rewarding to watch the development of voices among individuals who have been ignored in previous or traditional research processes.

PAR is the ultimate in social justice practice. I suggest that PAR should be the basis for all nursing research. This book will provide you with the basics for getting started. Good luck and enjoy!

Patricia J. Kelly, PhD, MPH, APRN
Professor, Associate Dean for Research, and
Coordinator of the PhD Program
School of Nursing and Health Studies
University of Missouri–Kansas City
Kansas City, Missouri

SERIES FOREWORD

In this section, which is published in all volumes of the series, we discuss some key aspects of any qualitative design. This is basic information that might be helpful to novice researchers or those new to the designs and methods described in each chapter. The material is not meant to be rigid and prescribed because qualitative research by its nature is fluid and flexible; the reader should use any ideas that are relevant and discard any ideas that are not relevant to the specific project in mind.

Before beginning a project, it is helpful to commit to publishing it. Of course, it will be publishable because you will use every resource at hand to make sure it is of high quality and contributes to knowledge. Theses and dissertations are meaningless exercises if only the student and committee know what was learned. It is rather heart-breaking to think of all the effort that senior faculty have exerted to complete a degree and yet not to have anyone else benefit by the work. Therefore, some additional resources are included here. Appendix A for each book is a list of journals that publish qualitative research. References to the current nursing qualitative research textbooks are included so that readers may find additional material from sources cited in those chapters.

FOCUS

In qualitative research the focus is emic—what we commonly think of as "from the participant's point of view." The researcher's point of view, called "the etic view," is secondary and does not take precedence over what the participant wants to convey, because in qualitative research, the focus is on the person and his or her story. In contrast, quantitative researchers take pains to learn as much as they can about a topic and focus the research data collection on what they want to know. Cases or subjects that do not provide information about the researcher's agenda are considered outliers and are discarded or treated as aberrant data. Qualitative researchers embrace outliers and actively seek diverse points of view from participants to enrich the data. They sample for diversity within groups and welcome different perceptions even if they seek fairly homogenous samples. For example, in Leenerts and Magilvy's (2000) grounded theory study to examine self-care practices among women, they narrowed the study to low-income, White, HIV-positive women but included both lesbian and heterosexual women.

PROPOSALS

There are many excellent sources in the literature on how to write a research proposal. A couple are cited here (Annersten, 2006; Mareno, 2012; Martin, 2010; Schmelzer, 2006), and examples are found in Appendices B, C, and D. Proposals for any type of research should include basic elements about the purpose, significance, theoretical support, and methods. What is often lacking is a thorough discussion about the rationale. The rationale is needed for the overall design as well as each step in the process. Why qualitative research? Why ethnography and not phenomenology? Why go to a certain setting? Why select the participants through word of mouth? Why use one particular type of software over another to analyze data?

Other common mistakes are not doing justice to significance and failure to provide sufficient theoretical support for the approach. In qualitative research, which tends to be theory generating instead of theory testing, the author still needs to explain why the study is conducted from a particular frame of reference. For example, in some ethnographic work, there are hypotheses that are tested based on the work of prior ethnographers who studied that culture, but there is still a need to generate new theory about current phenomena within that culture from the point of view of the specific informants for the subsequent study.

Significance is underappreciated as an important component of research. Without justifying the importance of the study or the potential impact of the study, there is no case for why the study should be conducted. If a study cannot be justified, why should sponsors fund it? Why should participants agree to participate? Why should the principal investigator bother to conduct it?

COMMONALITIES IN METHODS

Interviewing Basics

One of the best resources for learning how to interview for qualitative research is by Patton (2002), and readers are referred to his book for a detailed guide to interviewing. He describes the process, issues, and challenges in a way that readers can focus their interview in a wide variety of directions that are flexible, yet rigorous. For example, in ethnography, a mix of interview methods is appropriate, ranging from unstructured interviews or informal conversation to highly structured interviews. Unless nurses are conducting mixed-design studies, most of their interviews will be semistructured. Semistructured interviews include a few general questions, but the interviewer is free to allow the interviewee to digress along any lines he or she wishes. It is up to the interviewer to bring the interview back to the focus of the research. This requires skill and sensitivity.

Some general guidelines apply to semistructured interviews:

- Establish rapport.
- Ask open-ended questions. For example, the second question is much more likely to generate a meaningful response than the first in a grounded theory study of coping with cervical cancer.

    Interviewer: Were you afraid when you first heard your diagnosis of cervical cancer?

    Participant: Yes.

    Contrast the above with the following:

    Interviewer: What was your first thought when you heard your diagnosis of cervical cancer?

    Participant: I thought of my young children and how they were going to lose their mother and that they would grow up not knowing how much I loved them.

- Continuously "read" the person's reactions and adapt the approach based on response to questions. For example, in the interview about coping with the diagnosis, the participant began tearing so the interviewer appropriately gave her some time to collect herself. Maintaining silence is one of the most difficult things to learn for researchers who have been classically trained in quantitative methods. In structured interviewing, we are trained to continue despite distractions and to eliminate bias, which may involve eliminating emotion and emotional reactions to what we hear in the interview. Yet the quality of outcomes in qualitative designs may depend on the researcher–participant relationship. It is critical to be authentic and to allow the participant to be authentic.

Ethical Issues

The principles of the Belmont Commission apply to all types of research: respect, justice, beneficence. Perhaps these are even more important when interviewing people about their culture or life experiences. These are highly personal and may be painful for the person to relate, though I have found that there is a cathartic effect to participating in naturalistic research with an empathic interviewer (de Chesnay, 1991, 1993).

Rigor

Readers are referred to the classic paper on rigor in qualitative research (Sandelowski, 1986). Rather than speak of validity and reliability we use other terms, such as accuracy (Do the data represent truth as the participant sees it?) and replicability (Can the reader follow the decision trail to see why the researcher concluded as he or she did?).

DATA ANALYSIS

Analyzing data requires many decisions about how to collect data and whether to use high-tech measures such as qualitative software or old-school measures such as colored index cards. The contributors to this series provide examples of both.

Mixed designs require a balance between the assumptions of quantitative research while conducting that part and qualitative research during that phase. It can be difficult for novice researchers to keep things straight. Researchers are encouraged to learn each paradigm well and to be clear about why they use certain methods for their purposes. Each type of design can stand alone, and one should never think that qualitative research is *less than* quantitative; it is just different.

Mary de Chesnay

REFERENCES

Annersten, M. (2006). How to write a research proposal. *European Diabetes Nursing, 3*(2), 102–105.

de Chesnay, M. (1991, March 13–17). *Catharsis: Outcome of naturalistic research.* Presented to Society for Applied Anthropology, Charleston, SC.

de Chesnay, M. (1993). Workshop with Dr. Patricia Marshall of Symposium on Research Ethics in Fieldwork. Sponsored by Society for Applied Anthropology, Committee on Ethics. Memphis, March 25–29, 1992; San Antonio, Texas, March 11–14, 1993.

Leenerts, M. H., & Magilvy, K. (2000). Investing in self-care: A midrange theory of self-care grounded in the lived experience of low-income HIV-positive white women. *Advances in Nursing Science, 22*(3), 58–75.

Mareno, N. (2012). Sample qualitative research proposal: Childhood obesity in Latino families. In M. de Chesnay & B. Anderson (Eds.), *Caring for the vulnerable* (pp. 203–218). Sudbury, MA: Jones and Bartlett.

Martin, C. H. (2010). A 15-step model for writing a research proposal. *British Journal of Midwifery, 18*(12), 791–798.

Patton, M. Q. (2002). *Qualitative research and evaluation methods* (3rd ed.). Thousand Oaks, CA: Sage.

Sandelowski, M. (1986). The problem of rigor in qualitative research. *Advances in Nursing Science, 4*(3), 27–37.

Schmelzer, M. (2006). How to start a research proposal. *Gastroenterology Nursing, 29*(2), 186–188.

PREFACE

Qualitative research has evolved from a slightly disreputable beginning to wide acceptance in nursing research. Approaches that focus on the stories and perceptions of the people, instead of what scientists think the world is about, have been a tradition in anthropology for a long time and have created a body of knowledge that cannot be replicated in the lab. The richness of human experience is what qualitative research is all about. Respect for this tradition was long in coming among the scientific community. Nurses seem to have been in the forefront, and though many of my generation (children of the 1950s and 1960s) were classically trained in quantitative techniques, we found something lacking. Perhaps because I am a psychiatric nurse, I have been trained to listen to people tell me their stories, whether the stories are problems that nearly destroy the spirit, or uplifting accounts of how they live within their cultures, or how they cope with terrible traumas and chronic diseases. It seems logical to me that a critical part of developing new knowledge that nurses can use to help patients is to find out first what the patients themselves have to say.

In this volume, the focus is participatory action research (PAR). The chapter authors have made a point of providing the philosophical orientation to PAR as well as first-person accounts of their own studies. PAR is a type of method that should be quite comfortable for nurse researchers since we are accustomed to close interaction with communities. Advocating for patients is consistent with partnering with communities to accomplish health goals. Similarly, community leaders should be comfortable with nurse researchers who tend to give as much as they take when conducting research in communities. For example, our faculty at Duquesne University wanted to conduct research in the local poor community near the university, and in exchange for cooperation, the faculty taught CPR classes.

Other volumes address ethnography, grounded theory, life history, historical research, phenomenology, and data analysis. The volume on data analysis also includes material on focus groups and case studies, and two types of research that can be used with a variety of designs, including quantitative research and mixed designs. Efforts have been made to recruit contributors from several countries to demonstrate global applicability of qualitative research.

There are many fine textbooks on nursing research that provide an overview of all the methods, but our aim here is to provide specific information to guide graduate students and experienced nurses who are novices in the designs represented in this series in conducting studies from the point of view of our constituents—patients and their families. The studies conducted by contributors provide much practical advice for beginners as well as new ideas for experienced researchers. Some authors take a formal approach, but others speak quite personally in the first person. We hope you catch their enthusiasm and have fun conducting your own studies.

Mary de Chesnay

ACKNOWLEDGMENTS

In any publishing venture, there are many people who work together to produce the final draft. The contributors kindly share their expertise to offer advice and counsel to novices, and the reviewers ensure the quality of submissions. All of them have come up through the ranks as qualitative researchers and their participation is critical to helping novices learn the process.

No publication is successful without great people who not only know how to do their own jobs but also how to guide authors. At Springer Publishing Company, we are indebted to Margaret Zuccarini for the idea for the series, her ongoing support, and her excellent problem-solving skills. The person who guided the editorial process and was available for numerous questions, which he patiently answered as if he had not heard them a hundred times, was Joseph Morita. Also critical to the project were the people who proofed the work, marketed the series, and transformed it to hard copies, among them Jenna Vaccaro and Kris Parrish.

At Kennesaw State University, Dr. Tommie Nelms, Director of the WellStar School of Nursing, was a constant source of emotional and practical support in addition to her chapter contribution to the phenomenology volume. Her administrative assistant, Mrs. Cynthia Elery, kindly assigned student assistants to complete several chores, which enabled the author to focus on the scholarship. Bradley Garner, Chadwick Brown, and Chino Duke are our student assistants and unsung heroes of the university.

Finally, I am grateful to my cousin, Amy Dagit, whose expertise in proofreading saved many hours for some of the chapters.

If we are together, nothing is impossible.

—Winston Churchill

Chapter One

Participatory Action Research

Karen Lucas Breda

*I*f you are interested in helping to create meaningful change in a system or with a group of people, then you may want to read on. If you would like to find a method of research that genuinely involves the "subjects" in the research process, then you may want to read on. If you are looking for a research method that is collaborative and participatory and unlike most other forms of research, then you may want to read on. Participatory action research (PAR) does all of this and more.

PAR is a form of research that includes the research subjects in a meaningful way in every step of the research process. Research subjects are called "participants" in PAR because they are included as members of the team in every phase of the research process. The philosophy of PAR is that participants hold knowledge and are able to lend important advice and guidance to researchers. This democratizes the research process and radically changes the nature of the relationship between researchers and subjects.

The PAR methodology challenges almost all of our preconceptions about scientific research (especially concepts such as bias and objectivity). It turns what we thought we knew about the research process on its head, upside down and inside out. Some purely quantitative researchers have trouble understanding the participatory nature of PAR and may not consider it a legitimate method. Yet PAR is a form of research that is easily incorporated into existing programs and organizations. It can produce results that are highly efficacious, relevant, and sustainable.

Why conduct research to create change when it is possible to simply do projects to create change outside of the research process? All scientific research is systematic and has the ability to produce knowledge that can advance science. PAR can produce a unique type of knowledge that advances both the science and the discipline in which it is carried out. It is particularly relevant for the applied sciences and the social sciences where intricate human relationships are at stake. Nursing is a young science that can benefit from learning about and understanding as many forms of inquiry as possible. Only then can nurse researchers and scholars have a wide enough repertoire to choose the proper research methods for research problems and questions.

WHAT IS PAR?

PAR is a type of participatory and cooperative inquiry that has increased in popularity in the social sciences over the last 2 decades. As a methodology, PAR is holistic and egalitarian. As one of several methods under the rubric of "participatory inquiry," PAR stands out for its connection with political aspects of producing knowledge (Reason, 1994).

PAR is a highly practical, contemporary, and relevant form of research because it allows researchers not only to involve participants in every step of the research process but also to give them a voice and a meaningful role in the actions that emerge from the research study. PAR fits beautifully into the applied sciences and particularly into the discipline and science of nursing because of its holistic, collaborative, and applied nature. Many research problems relevant to nursing science involve the complexity of human behavior and straddle the boundaries of behavioral and social research. PAR is one of several action-oriented methodologies that can respond to research questions requiring social action and change. In recent years, PAR has taken hold in nursing and has grown considerably in popularity.

This chapter provides you with a brief history of PAR and guides you on the path of understanding how and when to use it. Chapter 2 of this volume treats the state of the art of PAR in nursing literature and explicates some of the groundbreaking ways nurse researchers have used this intriguing methodology.

THE ROOTS OF PAR

If you are thinking of using PAR in a research project or if you simply want to better appreciate it as a method, it is important to understand the background and evolution of the method. This section offers a snapshot of the philosophical underpinnings and historical roots of PAR. It also attempts to provide a lens into how one might conceptualize and implement a PAR project.

WHY AND WHERE DID PAR ORIGINATE?

Participatory forms of research allow the researcher to include the recipients of the research in the actual process of the research study. PAR is part of the broad category of approaches to participative inquiry that include (a) cooperative inquiry, (b) action science/action inquiry, and (c) PAR (Reason, 1994).

One way to understand PAR is to compare it to more traditional (sometimes called *orthodox*) forms of research. In the orthodox model of scientific research, the subjects of the research study are passive and have no formal role in the process other than being research subjects. In fact, great care is taken by orthodox researchers to distance themselves from the research subjects to remain as objective as possible and not to introduce bias or otherwise influence the findings of the study. Similarly, members of the community or the organization in which orthodox research is conducted are outside the research process and are not expected or even allowed to have an active role in the research study. Within the logic of orthodox science, this approach is logical and necessary for the research to proceed correctly. It gives the researcher control and authority of every aspect of the research process, and it gives the subject little control or authority. In orthodox research, subjects are fully informed and give consent to be studied, and they may withdraw from the study at any point, but they have little or no control or authority over how the research is conducted and carried out.

On the other hand, PAR finds its roots in a totally different philosophical reality. PAR does not follow the rules or format of orthodox science, and PAR researchers are not required to distance themselves from research subjects. Quite the opposite is true, in fact. PAR researchers are expected to break down the barriers between researcher and subject and to intentionally develop rapport and get to know the people who take part in the study. In participatory forms of research, the research subjects are referred to as participants because they actively participate in the entire process of the study. Orthodox research mandates that researchers distance themselves from research subjects. PAR (and other forms of participatory research) assumes, as Whyte, Greenwood, and Lazes maintain, that science "is not achieved by distancing oneself from the world; as generations of scientists know, the greatest conceptual and methodological challenges come from engagement with the world" (Whyte, Greenwood, & Lazes, 1991, p. 21).

PAR researchers engage in the world first and foremost by giving voice to study participants. Engagement begins when the researcher actively encourages participants from the beginning of the research process to play an active role. Whether the goal of PAR research is to reduce health disparities (Olshansky et al., 2005), enhance nursing autonomy (Breda et al., 2013), develop practice-based knowledge (Dampier, 2009), or improve care to those experiencing perinatal loss (Pastor-Montero et al., 2012), study participants have an active role in every phase of the research process. This engagement has a benefit to both researchers and participants. It allows researchers to get close to research participants, and it frees researchers from the need to remain distant and detached. At the same time, it allows participants to use their local knowledge about the issue to inform the research process and to increase its meaning and pertinence. In participatory forms of research, the philosophical stance is emancipating for both the researcher and the participant.

Another aspect of PAR is important to note. PAR has an essential and intentional political component. In fact, PAR requires the researcher to focus on the political aspects of producing knowledge (Breda et al., 2013). Not only does PAR acknowledge the role of power, it considers the ways in which knowledge is created. It pays attention to *who* holds power, *how* power is gained, *who* benefits from it, and vicariously, *who* is harmed or disadvantaged from the lack of power. This intentionally political dimension of PAR is a significant element that separates it from action research (AR).

Why did participatory forms of research emerge and why is it so different from orthodox science? The simple explanation is that researchers and scholars began to think that while orthodox science is important for many research questions and imperative to the development of scientific inquiry, particularly laboratory science, some research questions are not well addressed through orthodox scientific approaches. This different philosophical approach (sometimes called *new paradigm* science) planted the seeds for many of the qualitative research methodologies we use today and for many of the accompanying theories such as critical theory.

We answered the question *why* did PAR originate. Now it is time to consider *where* PAR originated because geographical location and philosophical traditions are intertwined. Location and philosophical traditions inform the method and explain why PAR varies slightly in different locations.

Northern Versus Southern PAR

PAR has two strands: one originated in the South, primarily in South America including Latin America and Brazil (PAR is called *investigación-acción participativa*, or IAP, in Spanish), and the other originated in the North, primarily in Anglo-North America (Schneider, 2012). The Southern strand of PAR emerged from a philosophy of critical theory and social action. Brazilian educator and philosopher Paolo Freire and Colombian critical sociologist Orlando Fals Borda are two leading figures in the development of the Southern strand of PAR. These architects of the Southern tradition of PAR sought social transformation and change as an integral part of the process. Southern PAR researchers looked to create projects with peasants, workers, disabled persons, people from ethnic minorities, and others who are oppressed and exploited by political, economic, and class circumstances.

Over time, Fals Borda and his Southern PAR research team in Colombia, South America, attracted international scholars who wanted to learn more about the method. Some of them were anthropologists and sociologists while others came from diverse applied fields. Initially teachers, agronomists, and veterinarians became interested, and later "with the periodic regional and world congresses physicians, dentists, nurses, social economists and engineers approached" (Fals Borda, 2013, p. 158). Still later, historians, humanists, musicians, and even mathematicians were drawn to Southern PAR as a methodology they could embrace. Ethnomathematics, the main concern of which was to "improve teaching schemes to render them less frightening to young people," was developed as an alternative way to teach mathematics (p. 158).

Simultaneously in Brazil, Paolo Freire developed a PAR project with poor peasants who were unable to read. He developed an alternative educational strategy called *educação popular* (Portugese) and *educación popular* (in Spanish). In English the terms *popular education* or *critical education* are used (originally, but no longer translated as "adult education") to refer to Freire's view of teaching using alternative teaching formats with the intention of creating a critical awakening as well as new knowledge (Freire, 1996a, 1996b, www.popednews.org). Freire wrote about this form of teaching literacy, calling it "education for critical consciousness." In writing about this experience, Freire explained that he and participants working with him tried to "design a project in which we would attempt to move from naïveté to a critical attitude at the same time we taught reading" (1996b, p. 42).

The goal of Freire's literacy project was to work with those who were marginalized and disempowered in society to help them to gain an understanding of their circumstances and to become aware of the need to create social change. Rather than teach them to read using the traditional "banking" method, Freire used PAR to empower the group to help develop a strategy that allowed them to teach each other to read. For example, the peasants were not able to read leases and other legal documents. Prior to learning to read, they could be tricked into signing things they did not understand. Working with the PAR literacy project gave them the ability to read and to advocate for themselves and others. As a result, in addition to acquiring the knowledge to learn to read, they gained power, awareness, and a critical consciousness (Freire, 1996b).

These Southern PAR pioneers, Orlando Fals Borda and Paolo Freire, were contemporaries—both were born in the 1920s. They viewed PAR as more than a methodology. In their eyes, PAR was part of a movement that included a new way of thinking and doing science. Before doing a PAR study, they believed that researchers had to change their own way of thinking and that it was not possible for strict orthodox researchers to engage in Southern PAR because it requires a critical stance that is philosophically opposed to conventional, orthodox science. In essence, they wanted PAR research to create meaningful change in both the social and cultural contexts as well as in the scientific realm (Fals Borda, 2013).

Fals Borda worked within existing structures of autonomous institutions such as the Rosca Foundation and aligned himself with progressive political parties, while Freire worked within critical movements connected to labor unions of teachers (Fals Borda, 2013, p. 163). Both intellectuals immersed themselves in their communities of interest and took a path of civic resistance rather than militancy. By necessity, Southern PAR is linked to political activism and involvement and to the quest for social justice and societal transformation.

The Northern tradition of PAR developed earlier and in a different way than the Southern strand. Northern PAR is less radical and less political than Southern PAR, and more overlap exists between action research (AR) and PAR in the North. Most reports link psychologist Kurt Lewin to the development of the Northern version of PAR because he was the first to use the term AR. For those interested in the timeline for PAR development, Kurt Lewin (1890–1947) lived and worked before the time of Fals Borda and Paolo Freire.

Kurt Lewin was a pioneer in social and organizational psychology, and he is known, above all, for his change theory. He developed "a practical approach to problem solving through a cycle of planning, action, and reflection" (Schneider, 2012, p. 154). He worked in industrial settings to try to create more democratic workplaces and has influenced the literature on workplace organization and what recently has been called "collaborative improvement processes" (p. 154).

Kurt Lewin had a fascinating career. A Prussian Jew born in 1890, Lewin had a background in social justice and social transformation. His family moved to Germany, where he attended university and studied psychology. He associated with the left-leaning Frankfurt School, was involved in the socialist movement and in women's rights. He immigrated to the United States in 1933, the same year that Hitler came to power in Germany. In the United States, he turned his interests to Gestalt psychology, sensitivity training, and later coined the term *action research*.

Lewin believed that research should have a purpose beyond that of producing scholarly articles and books. For him, research should lead to social action. Focusing on the need to improve intergroup relations, Lewin attempted to understand the role of attitudes and stereotypes as well as the influence social class, politics, and economics had on behavior. Lewin was a social psychologist and as such he was interested in learning how to change social behavior. His three step theory of change (Unfreeze–Change–Refreeze) is known worldwide.

The Northern strand of PAR strives both for advancing human knowledge and improving welfare (Whyte et al., 1991). It includes, among other things, studies in industry and agriculture. One example of PAR in industry is a study of union workers at New York State's Xerox Corporation, another is a study of the FAGOR group of worker cooperatives in the Basque area of Spain, and a third example is the study of quality circle programs in U.S. companies. An example of PAR in agriculture is a study of third world development and small farmers.

Whether one adheres to the Northern or Southern tradition of PAR, it is important to know when PAR is a good choice to use as a methodology. The next section explores how and when to use PAR, and hopefully this information will help you decide if PAR is a good method to use in a future study.

HOW AND WHEN TO USE PAR

If your research problem entails a group of people who are marginalized, exploited, or in some way disempowered, consider using PAR. PAR is appropriate to adopt as a method when issues exist concerning ownership of knowledge and where the need exists "to create communities of people who are capable of continuing the PAR process" (Reason, in Denzin & Lincoln, 1994, p. 335). It is a suitable form of research to use in areas where the gap between the rich and poor is great and in marginalized communities where political issues concerning ownership of knowledge are apparent. PAR might be successful when you, as the researcher, are willing to allow the research participants a role "in setting the agendas, participating in the data gathering and analysis, and controlling the use of the outcomes" (p. 329).

With PAR, additional time is needed to get to know the community, to develop rapport, to learn the local norms, to find key informants, and to be sure that research participants are able to involve themselves in a long-term effort. The methodology of PAR can entail the use of either quantitative or qualitative methods or both. This will be determined by the nature of the research problem and the most fitting way to answer the research questions. Peter Reason (1994) points to a variety of activities that can constitute a PAR research project. Reason writes that:

> Community meetings and events of various kinds are an important part of PAR, serving to identify issues, to reclaim a sense of community and emphasize the potential for liberation, to make sense of information collected, to reflect on the progress of the project, and to develop the ability of the community to continue the PAR and developmental process. (p. 329)

Activities and interventions, usually not associated with orthodox research, are often a part of the PAR process. Photography, artistic endeavors, poetry, music, theater, performance, dance, role playing, games, team building, workshops, and experiential education are a few ways PAR engages participants. Activities are not chosen haphazardly. The activity is chosen because it fits not only the objective of the research, but also the culture and environment of the participants.

PAR is as much a way of doing research as it is a method of research. It is a philosophy, as well as a research method. It is not doing research on subjects but doing research with participants. PAR participants guide the researcher to discover the research question. Researchers are the experts in academic knowledge, but participants are the "experts" in local knowledge. Academic knowledge and local knowledge are used equally to design a plan. Participants guide researchers with their local knowledge and together they co-create a feasible intervention plan. Reflection and evaluation are also joint activities between researchers and participants. Adult education, also called "popular education," is often adopted in PAR as a way of learning together. Giving voice to research participants allows PAR researchers to better understand the issues from the participants' points of view and to develop action-oriented interventions that benefit the community.

Phases of PAR

How to do PAR is more difficult to understand than why to do PAR. The philosophical roots of PAR are clear and well documented in the literature.

However, the steps or phases of the PAR process are less well defined and reported. The iterative process of PAR methodology is the most important feature to keep in mind. This means that the steps or phases of PAR are cyclical and dynamic. It is possible and even desirable to repeat the steps again and again, increasing in complexity and understanding with each cycle.

The processes of establishing rapport, planning, action, reflection, and evaluation are generally considered to be the basic steps of the PAR process. Others break the PAR process into eight phases, adding steps such as goal setting, identification of team members, finding funding, and data analysis. This type of conceptualization is inherently linear with mutually exclusive phases or steps. Consequently, it deters one from thinking in a cyclical or dynamic fashion. Using the conceptualization of establishing rapport, planning, action, reflection, and evaluation serves as a useful guide to both novice and expert researchers. It helps to keep them on track and not to leave out any of the essential components, while allowing for the iterative and cyclical nature of PAR.

SUMMARY AND CONCLUSIONS

PAR is a fascinating and powerful methodology to advance practice and science (Whyte et al., 1991). Because it involves the research subjects (called "participants" in the PAR framework) in every step of the research process, it forces researchers to take into account multiple points of view and, particularly, the worldview of the "other." It turns conventional research methodology on its head, and it challenges us at every corner to rethink our deep-seated bias and preconceptions stemming from the orthodox research process. PAR is a holistic, egalitarian methodology producing results that are relevant, practical, and sustainable. It fits perfectly into nursing and is a good addition to the repertoire of methods used by applied nurse scientists.

PAR is considered new paradigm science. It stems philosophically from a range of critical theories, such as neo-Marxist, post-colonial, and feminist theories. PAR can be loosely divided into a more radical Southern strand and a less radical Northern strand. Southern PAR researchers generally work with disenfranchised and marginalized groups and communities using methods such as participatory popular education (adult education), artistic endeavors, and consciousness building. The goal is for action and social transformation aiming ultimately for social justice and equal rights. Northern PAR researchers generally work in industry and with occupational groups on workplace issues. The assumption is that labor and management "can work together to create more democratic workplaces" (Schneider, 2012, p. 154). The goal is for action and improved collaborative relationships and enhanced workplace teams.

PAR is best used with exploited and disenfranchised groups of people, where gaps in knowledge and equal rights are large and where the hope for empowerment is the greatest. Understanding the political dimensions of who holds power, how power is exercised, and who is harmed or disadvantaged by power is integral to the PAR process. It is this political dimension that distinguishes PAR from AR.

PAR researchers engage with participants in their local environments and cultures. Target populations for PAR researchers may be groups exposed to alcohol, drugs, domestic violence, and other forms of abuse; groups with disabilities; or groups suffering from ethnic, racial, and class exploitation. Oppressed women, teens, and those with chronic diseases and physical and mental illnesses are also included. Additionally, PAR researchers may choose to work with professionals, semiprofessionals, labor unionists, agricultural workers, undocumented workers, migrant workers, sex workers, persons who are homeless or at risk for homelessness, immigrant groups, and people living in conflict or war zones. This is a partial list of potential target populations for PAR methodology.

The nature of the research problem and the focus of the research help to determine the type of methodology that is suitable. Qualitative or quantitative methods can be used in PAR. Additional time is needed in PAR research to develop rapport and to build community among participants. The steps of the PAR process are generally agreed to be establishing rapport, planning, action, reflection, and evaluation. They are dynamic in nature and are also called iterative, meaning that they are repetitive and cyclical rather than linear in nature.

Participants are considered to be the holders of local knowledge in PAR research. In fact, one of the main goals of PAR is to be useful to the people (Reason, 1994). This is done through activities such as community building meetings, consciousness-raising encounters including but not limited to artistic endeavors, adult/popular education, drama, poetry, workshops, training, and so on. A second goal of PAR is "to empower people at a second and deeper level through the process of constructing and using their own knowledge" (p. 328). Oppressed and exploited groups are often unaware of their own knowledge. They may feel shame and humiliation at their own condition (e.g., mental illness, disability, poverty, substance abuse) and, in this state, they are unable to recognize the value and authenticity of their own local knowledge, know-how, and expertise.

PAR has a strong alternative philosophical foundation that influences it as a research methodology. Research participants become research partners in the PAR process. Doing research with participants is not a good fit for every research scientist, and one should consider this closely prior to engaging in PAR. PAR studies are carried out best by researchers who understand its collaborative and egalitarian elements. Also, research problems that align well with the PAR philosophy are easier to implement and ultimately more successful in accomplishing goals. PAR can be a labor-intensive methodology. Many PAR researchers find it a professionally rewarding method to use, and they choose the method for the humanistic and transformational sociopolitical rewards it can generate.

In closing, PAR is a dynamic methodology relevant to 21st-century nurses and other applied social scientists. Learning about this fascinating methodology and advocating its appropriate use can help expand both the science and discipline of nursing.

REFERENCES

Breda, K. L. (2013). Critical ethnography. In C. T. Beck (Ed.), *Routledge international handbook of qualitative nursing research* (pp. 230–241). New York, NY: Routledge.

Dampier, S. (2009). Action research. *Nurse researcher, 16*(2), 4.

Fals Borda, O. (2013). Action research in the convergence of disciplines. *International Journal of Action Research, 9*(2), 155–167.

Freire, P. (1996a). *Pedagogy of the oppressed.* New York, NY: Continuum.

Freire, P. (1996b). *Education for critical consciousness.* New York, NY: Continuum.

Olshansky, D. S., Braxter, B., Dodge, P., Hughes, E., Ondeck, M., Stubbs, M., & Upvall, M. (2005). Participatory action research to understand and reduce health disparities. *Nursing Outlook 53*(3), 121–126.

Pastor-Montero, S. M., Romero-Sánchez, J. M., Paramio-Cuevas, J. C., Hueso-Montoro, C., Paloma-Castro, O., Lillo-Crespo, M., . . . Frandsen, A. J. (2012). Tackling perinatal loss, a participatory action research approach: Research protocol. *Journal of Advanced Nursing, 68*(11), 2578–2585.

Reason, P. (1994). Three approaches to participatory inquiry. In N. Denzin & Y. Lincoln (Eds.), *Handbook of qualitative research* (pp. 324–339). Thousand Oaks, CA: Sage.

Schneider, B. (2012). Participatory action research: Mental health service user research, and the hearing (our) voices projects. *International Journal of Qualitative Methods, 11*(2), 152–165. The Popular Education News. Retrieved from www.popednews.org

Whyte, W. F., Greenwood, D. J., & Lazes, P. (1991). Participatory action research: Through practice to science in social research. In W. F. Whyte (Ed.), *Participatory Action Research* (pp. 19–55). Newbury Park, CA: Sage.

Chapter Two

State of the Art of Nursing Research in Participatory Action Research

Karen Lucas Breda

Over the past 15 years, participatory action research (PAR) has become increasingly popular in health science research. Nursing is part of this trend. PAR is often used to study issues related to social justice and oppression with disenfranchised groups. Inequities pertaining to health status as well as ethnic, racial, and class disparities in health are some of the concerns dear to nursing that can be appropriately addressed using PAR. While PAR is often cited as an ideal methodology for studying inequity, oppression, and injustice, PAR methodology is also highly suitable for the study of organizations, organization change, work life, and the dynamics of occupational and professional groups. The purpose of this chapter is to highlight key PAR studies conducted in nursing and the contribution PAR has made to nursing science.

PAR STUDIES CONDUCTED BY NURSES

This section looks chronologically at work done by nursing using PAR. It is not all-inclusive. Rather, it attempts to capture key studies that are indicative of a variety of population groups and topics studied. It also describes some nursing studies using action research (AR) to give the flavor of topics appropriate for AR. Basic differences between AR and PAR are pointed out.

Breda and colleagues (1997) used PAR to study professional autonomy with a group of nurses at a small, rural psychiatric hospital. Through the PAR process, autonomy emerged as the single most important issue for the nurses, even more than salary and benefits. The study followed an earlier ethnographic study by Breda (1997) in the same facility that examined how nurses worked together in a labor union to promote their status as professionals in the hospital. The earlier ethnographic study allowed Breda to develop rapport and trusting relationships with nurses and other caregivers in the facility. The subsequent PAR study was a natural product of the ethnographic study. Conducting ethnography opened the doors for using PAR as a participatory and action-oriented form of inquiry. The PAR study allowed the nurses to have meaningful input into a reflective process for change, and the process had a positive impact on nursing practice for the participants.

Dickson and Green (2001) conducted a PAR study with Aboriginal grandmothers in Canada. The authors defined PAR as "inquiry by ordinary people acting as researchers to explore questions in their daily lives, to recognize their own resources, and to produce knowledge and take action to overcome inequities, often in solidarity with external supporters" (p. 472). With this method in mind the authors worked with 40 Aboriginal grandmothers from remote rural areas to generate knowledge and to empower participants. Some of this involved the grandmothers developing a sense of well-being that entailed "learning other coping skills, establishing new social support systems, and reclaiming their traditional role as sources of wisdom, guidance, and love" (p. 473).

The purpose of the PAR project was to study the health needs of the grandmothers and to respond to those needs through health promotion programs. In light of the oppression and exploitation of Aboriginal people in Canada, and central to PAR methodology, researchers were acutely aware of the need to give voice to the grandmothers. The PAR process allowed participants to create activities for healing and personal development, to be aware of their own strengths, and to build self-esteem. Weekly gatherings over a prolonged period of time helped them build knowledge, self-confidence, community, and sisterhood. After solidarity grew, they began to advocate for themselves and the larger Aboriginal community.

Olshansky and colleagues (2005) reported on several PAR studies connected to the goal of reducing health disparities. Nurse researchers in each study worked collaboratively with community members to create research partnerships. The ultimate goal was to create "constructive social change" toward the goal of reducing health disparities (p. 123). Upvall worked with Somali refugees in the United States. The intention was that the PAR study would provide "the foundation for community programs and the development of handbooks necessary for guiding resettlement efforts" (Olshansky et al., 2005, p. 124). Dodge, Hughes, and Ondeck (in Olshansky et al., 2005) designed a community outreach program focused on minority health. The "Families in Motion" and the "Walking DIVAs" programs were developed to address the increased risk African American women have for diabetes and obesity. The groups walk together for "physical activity and social support" (p. 125). African American women in "Families in Motion" were able to successfully implement a walking program "to contribute to improved health" (p. 123). The co-researchers then developed subsequent interventions including a "train the trainer" component. Using successful PAR outcomes to shape subsequent interventions allowed researchers to grow and refine the program. This *iterative* or repetitive process is characteristic of PAR. It means that researchers dip back into all of the phases of the research using a reflective process to revise and expand interventions.

In 2006, University of British Columbia Professor Colleen Varcoe published a paper reflecting on her use of PAR as a method in more than four major studies. In the paper titled "Doing PAR in a Racist World" Vancoe describes her use of a critical antiracist framework in studies focusing on the power dynamics of race. She explicates the strengths and weaknesses of PAR when studying sensitive topics such as racism, violence, and sexual abuse.

Varcoe (2006) critiques her position of power and privilege vis-à-vis her study participants and struggles with her role as the principal researcher. She describes her challenges with not being able to recruit and retain women of color and Aboriginal women as study participants. In one study on the topic of intimate partner violence (IPV), she added a dimension of role confusion by sharing with participants that she herself had suffered IPV. In another project, some of the research participants became angry with a perceived racist agenda and walked off the research project. The staff on her team reviewed the behavioral and racist messages they might have been sending (albeit inadvertently) to participants. The team revised study protocols for the future, keeping in mind the delicate nature of race and class relations in an advanced capitalist society. Varcoe (2006) explains the ambiguous role of the PAR researcher aptly when she writes "[if] nurse researchers (and those from other disciplines) want to engage in empowering research, they ought to expect to get overpowered once in a while" (p. 538).

The issues pertaining to researcher–participant relationships bring to the fore the sticky business of qualitative research, including reflexivity, and in the case of PAR, the even more intimate role of the researcher in the lives of the participants. PAR carries with it the need for researchers to be comfortable maintaining a high level of transparency with participants. Also, for true collaboration to exist, participants will want to critique as well as participate in the PAR process.

Fals Borda (2013) gives us a philosophical direction in these matters. He calls for PAR researchers to first change themselves and to relinquish control to the participants and to the community. In the process of doing PAR, he discovered that science and knowledge generation is not something reserved for elite intellectuals in academic settings. "The scientific spirit" according to Fals Borda "can flourish under the most modest and primitive of circumstances, that important work is not necessarily expensive or complicated, nor must it become a monopoly of a class or the academia" (p. 161). This stance led to an authenticity of the researcher to the subject and what Fals Borda called "authentic participation," where academic knowledge and popular knowledge are both considered valuable and have meaning (p. 160).

Research nurses Etowa, Bernard, Oyinsan, and Clow (2007) used PAR in their attempt to improve Black women's health in rural and remote communities in Canada. Black Nova Scotians suffer from dramatic social and health inequities even though they have inhabited the area for centuries and make up "one of the largest indigenous visible minorities in the country" (p. 349). Authors developed a community–academic collaborative PAR project, called "on the margins" (OTM), with Black Nova Scotians focusing on health status and health system use. The study used an interdisciplinary team from nursing, women's studies, social work, and women's health to partner with participants in the community who were trained as community research facilitators.

The team was acutely aware of the need to give voice to the co-researchers and to foster knowledge generation in their PAR project. Recognizing that one goal of PAR is to engender empowerment and transformation through "capacity building to effect change" (Etowa et al., 2007, p. 351), the authors struggled with the challenges of PAR, realizing that simply forming partnerships with the community does not automatically guarantee empowerment and transformation. One of the broad concerns pertaining to PAR methodology is that some researchers give lip service to the principles of participation, collaboration, and inclusion of participants in knowledge generation and the direction of the research without relinquishing any control. Constraints related to the time frame of research projects in light of funding schedules, the need to publish, and the overarching demands of tenure and promotion may either preclude researchers from using PAR or push them to take short cuts by engaging in nominal rather than substantial collaboration and inclusion of participants. This issue is part of the wider discourse concerning all forms of participatory research outside of nursing. Now, these discussions are taking a prominent place in the nursing literature as well.

Several nursing research studies from Spain inform our understanding on how PAR is used in that country. Abad-Corpa and colleagues (2010) published an article describing their intent to use a PAR design to study the effectiveness of the implementation of an evidence-based nursing model in oncohemotology. The intent of the researchers was to use a mixed-method approach to introduce a model of change for clinical practice in oncology. The authors used the soft systems methodology (SSM) of British scholar Peter Checkland in their study. Checkland worked in industry and developed a problem-solving method for the workplace that follows a step-by-step process for collaborative and participatory problem solving.

Another interesting PAR study planned to be carried out in Spain will look at perinatal loss. Pastor-Montero and colleagues (2012) aim to promote changes to improve the care provided to parents who have experienced a perinatal loss. They will follow the PAR process and use it together with focus groups, and a SWOT (strengths, weaknesses, opportunities, and threats) analysis. The authors see the PAR process as a spiral that is "reminiscent of the nursing process" (p. 2580). The PAR work is influenced by Fals Borda and the Southern strand and will follow five stages: "outreach and awareness, induction, interaction, implementation, and systematization" (Pastor-Montero et al., 2012, p. 2580).

Research nurse and anthropologist Travers-Gustafson and social worker Iluebbey (2013) compared the concepts of "traditional discipline" with "domestic violence" in a fascinating study carried out with a Sudanese refugee community residing in the United States. The collaborative nature of PAR allowed the authors to approach the delicate topic of this research and to explore experiences of resettlement, danger and role relationship changes, family conflict, and domestic violence within the context of the U.S. legal system. The study focused specifically on the issue of "*traditional discipline* as a form of domestic and intimate partner violence" (Travers-Gustafson & Iluebbey, 2013, p. 51).

There are dramatically different cultural understandings and role expectations for husbands and wives: In Sudan, husbands are legally permitted to hit or beat their wives, whereas in the United States, husbands hitting or beating their wives is defined as "domestic violence" and considered a crime. Both Sudanese women and men were surprised to know that a man could go to jail for hitting or beating his wife in the United States. In Sudan, a good husband was expected to beat his wife if she did not obey him or failed to perform household chores to his level of expectation. The Sudanese considered the practice of husbands hitting wives "traditional discipline" and not a crime.

After conducting separate focus groups with men and women and exploring the role of Sudanese elders in the refugee community, the authors arranged a series of community meetings using the PAR process that included both refugee and nonrefugee communities as well as law enforcement and health and social services providers. The purpose of the community meetings was to open dialogue and to educate all of the constituents. For example, U.S. police officers, social workers, and nurses viewed physical violence in black-and-white terms—it was always a crime. Sudanese wives were frightened of having their husbands in jail because it left them alone to care for their households. Often, it meant losing their source of income and their means of transportation as usually only Sudanese husbands drove. Husbands felt humiliated when arrested and confused about what it was that they did wrong.

The PAR-inspired community meetings led to the identification of a team of respected Sudanese elders made up of both men and women. After negotiations with law enforcement, a plan was made to train the team of Sudanese elders to identify domestic violence and allow the elders to be the mediators to Sudanese wives and husbands to help them settle disputes and "to prevent potential violence, injury and incarceration" (p. 55). Additional follow-up and an action plan were put in place with scheduled times for periodic reviews and refinements. Sudanese wives, husbands, and elders were given a voice in the process, and a concerted effort was made to have them partner with social service, health, and law enforcement representatives. In this successful PAR study, community members worked together to share knowledge and to create an individualized community plan for advocacy and change. The goal of maintaining community cohesiveness while addressing crucial role relationship changes, family conflict, and resettlement issues was achieved. Ongoing and "engaged problem solving and policy development" was a critical aspect of the PAR agenda to keep lines of communication open and to maintain success after the study was complete (p. 56). Funding issues for the future were recognized as a limitation.

This study is a model of how PAR can be used to "understand and improve the world by changing it" (Baum, MacDougall, & Smith, 2006, p. 854). Practicing nurses, social workers, and other service providers often generalize about the behavior of groups and, in the case of domestic violence, often advocate for extreme measures that can break up families and dissolve community cohesiveness. This research demonstrates that PAR as an example of a "new paradigm science" can use embedded local knowledge to create both action and change for social transformation, to build community cohesiveness, and to redirect patterns of behavior.

Canadian nurse researcher and anthropologist Karen Clements (2012) explored the concept of recovery among individuals experiencing mental illness in the project "Our Photos, Our Voices." Working within an empowerment recovery framework, she used PAR together with a method called *photovoice* to explore recovery using the personal experiences of a group who frequented a community psychosocial rehabilitation center called the

"Clubhouse" in Winnipeg, Canada. This collaborative mental health research project was intended to explore, document, share, and disseminate local knowledge about recovery as understood by persons experiencing mental illness. While the pilot project reported in the article is small, the combination of methodologies used proved to be an effective way of eliciting valuable stories and narratives from this population.

The empowerment recovery framework challenges conventional notions of mental illness and psychiatry. "Reclaiming one's own story" is an important component of allowing persons living with mental illness to define the meaning of their personal experiences. Health care professionals have long held the prerogative to define mental illness including the concepts of "cure" and "recovery" (Clements, 2012, p. 786). Allowing individuals experiencing mental illness to "envision recovery on one's own terms" allows them to recoup a higher level of power and self-determination.

Photovoice is a research methodology that uses photographs taken by research participants "to illustrate their ideas, their concerns and the realities of their lives" (p. 787). It has many elements in common with PAR and like PAR it emanates from the work of the Brazilian educator Paolo Freire. Clements's selection of PAR and photovoice is a masterful combination of complementary methodologies. Both PAR and photovoice allow participants to construct their own knowledge. In PAR the knowledge and experience of people, "often oppressed groups—is directly honored and valued" (Reason, 1994, p. 328). Not only does photovoice consider people the experts in their own lives (even persons experiencing mental illness or other disabilities), but it also facilitates a "critical awareness of issues important to the community, and support[s] community members in identifying problems and potential solutions" (Clements, 2012, p. 787). Fortunately, the researchers plan to continue using these methods and exploring the meaning of recovery in the Clubhouse "Our Photos, Our Voices" project. The ultimate test of success will be the social transformation and change that takes place not only at the Clubhouse but also in the wider community and territory.

ACTION RESEARCH

In addition to PAR studies, nurses have engaged in numerous research projects using AR. AR projects are participatory in nature. However, usually they do not link to the broader political context. While we do not fully review or critique AR projects carried out by nurses in this chapter, the following section gives some examples of studies well worth exploring.

Critical AR was used to develop clinical placements in aged-care facilities for undergraduate nursing students undertaking their nursing practicum topics. Xiao, Kelton, and Paterson's goal was to increase interest in elder nursing care among the new generation of nursing students (2011). Seib, English, and Barnard (2011) used AR to develop, deliver, and evaluate the community health nursing curriculum in an undergraduate nursing program. The goal was to increase students' engagement and learning in the course.

AR is considered a very useful and beneficial research method to reflect on, change, and advance nursing practice. The following AR projects address nursing practice issues. Reed (2005) used AR in nursing practice with older people in an attempt to develop practice-based knowledge and in general to democratize knowledge for this vulnerable population.

Lakeman and Glasgow (2009) used AR to introduce peer-group clinical supervision to psychiatric nurses in Trinidad. The goal was to enable practicing nurses to develop professional leadership and mentoring skills in a cost-effective manner. Researchers Gaudine, Gien, Thuan, and Dung (2009) used an AR approach to develop culturally sensitive interventions for health issues considered important to a Vietnamese community. Similarly, Jones, Auton, Burton, and Watkins (2008) and members of the local stroke community identified and prioritized service issues. Their goal was to develop local stroke services by genuinely involving those affected by stroke. Ryan and Happell (2009) conducted an AR study to discover the needs of hospitalized psychiatric patients after seclusion (with physical or chemical restraints). Post-seclusion debriefing practices between mental health nurses and patients were studied and revised based on the findings.

An AR approach was used to develop nurses' abilities to reflect on how to create good caring relationships with patients in palliative care. The results of this study conducted by Bergdahl, Benzein, Ternestedt, and Andershed (2011) showed that AR can help to develop emerging theory around caring. These examples are merely a selection of studies and do not represent a complete account of existing AR by nurses.

SUMMARY

This chapter introduced you to a complement of PAR studies in nursing. It addressed the state of the art of PAR in nursing literature and explicated some of the innovative ways nurse researchers are using this exciting methodology.

REFERENCES

Abad-Corpa, E., Meseguer-Liza, C., Martínez-Corbalán, J. T., Zárate-Riscal, L., Caravaca-Hernandez, A., Paredes-Sidrach de Cardona, A., . . . Cabrero-García, J. (2010). Effectiveness of the implementation of an evidence-based nursing model using participatory action research in oncohematology: Research protocol. *Journal of Advanced Nursing, 66*(8), 1845–1851.

Baum, F., MacDougall, C., & Smith, D. (2006). Participatory action research. *Journal of Epidemiology & Community Health, 60*, 854–857.

Bergdahl, E., Benzein, E., Ternestedt, B. M., & Andershed, B. (2011). Development of nurses' ability to reflect on how to create good caring relationships with patients in palliative care: An action research approach. *Nursing Inquiry, 18*(2), 111–122.

Breda, K. L. (1997). Professional nurses in unions: Working together pays off. *Journal of Professional Nursing, 13*(2), 99–109.

Breda, K. L., Anderson, M. A., Hansen, L., Hayes, D., Pillion, C., & Lyon, P. (1997). Enhanced nursing autonomy through participatory action research. *Nursing Outlook, 45*(2), 76–81.

Clements, K. (2012). Participatory action research and photovoice in a psychiatric nursing/clubhouse collaboration exploring recovery narrative. *Journal of Psychiatric and Mental Health Nursing, 19*, 785–791.

Dickson, G., & Green, K. L. (2001). Participatory action research: Lessons learned with aboriginal grandmothers. *Health Care for Women International, 22*, 471–482.

Etowa, J. B., Bernard, W. T., Oyinsan, B., & Clow, B. (2007). Participatory Action Research (PAR): An approach for improving black women's health in rural and remote communities. *Journal of Transcultural Nursing, 18*(4), 349–357.

Fals Borda, O. (2013). Action research in the convergence of disciplines. *International Journal of Action Research, 9*(2), 155–167.

Gaudine, A., Gien, L., Thuan, T. T., & Dung, D. V. (2009). Developing cultural sensitive interventions for Vietnamese health issues: An action research approach. *Nursing and Health Sciences, 11*, 150–153.

Jones, S. P., Auton, M. F., Burton, C. R., & Watkins, C. L. (2008). Engaging service users in the development of stroke services: An action research study. *Journal of Clinical Nursing, 17*(10), 1270–1279.

Lakeman, R., & Glasgos, C. (2009). Introducing peer-group clinical supervision: An action research project. *International Journal of Mental Health Nursing, 18*(3), 204–210.

Olshansky, D. S., Braxter, B., Dodge, P., Hughes, E., Ondeck, M., Stubbs, M., & Upvall, M. (2005). Participatory action research to understand and reduce health disparities. *Nursing Outlook, 53*(3), 121–126.

Pastor-Montero, S. M., Romero-Sánchez, J. M., Paramio-Cuevas, J. C., Hueso-Montoro, C., Paloma-Castro, O., Lillo-Crespo, M., . . . Frandsen, A. J. (2012). Tackling perinatal loss, a participatory action research approach: Research protocol. *Journal of Advanced Nursing, 68*(11), 2578–2585.

Reason, P. (1994). Three approaches to participatory inquiry. In N. K. Denzin & Y. S. Lincoln (Eds.), *Handbook of qualitative research* (pp. 324–339). Thousand Oaks, CA: Sage.

Reed, J. (2005). Using action research with older people: Democratizing knowledge. *Journal of Clinical Nursing, 14*(5), 594–600.

Ryan, R., & Happell, B. (2009). Learning from experience: Using action research to discover consumer needs in post-seclusion debriefing. *International Journal of Mental Health Nursing, 18*(2), 100–107.

Seib, C., English, R., & Barnard, A. (2011). Teaching undergraduate students community nursing: Using action research to increase engagement and learning. *Journal of Nursing Education, 50*(9), 537–539.

Travers-Gustafson, D., & Iluebbey, V. (2013). "Traditional discipline" or domestic violence: Participatory action research with a Sudanese refugee community. *Journal of Cultural Diversity, 20*(2), 1–56.

Varcoe, C. (2006). Doing participatory action research in a racist world. *Western Journal of Nursing Research, 28*(5), 525–540.

Xiao, L. D., Kelton, M., & Paterson, J. (2011). Critical action research applied in clinical placement development in aged care facilities. *Nursing Inquiry, 19*(4), 322–333.

CHAPTER THREE

PARTICIPATORY ACTION RESEARCH PROCEDURES

Anne Watson Bongiorno

The goal of this chapter is to provide a guide for structuring participatory action research (PAR) and to explore its theoretical underpinnings. PAR is not a research method but an emancipatory approach to inquiry, where the subjects are also the collaborators. The mindset of researchers needs to include a boldness of spirit, a quest for inclusiveness, shared power, and democracy in the research process.

PAR is rooted in traditions that empower oppressed communities to engage in critical analysis of evidence and to develop action for social change (Simonds & Christopher, 2013; Williamson, Bellman, & Webster, 2012). The approach starts with an understanding of the community of interest as the authoritative expert in its own life experience. PAR builds a culturally competent and cooperative partnership with the community of interest as an inherent part of the research itself (D'Alonzo, 2010).

The steps of PAR are to develop a co-generative dialogue with the community of interest through immersion and problem identification, to decide on a research strategy and process, and to use joint, critical analysis as a basis to enact change (Whyte, 1991). The community as expert provides vital context regarding findings. The stages of PAR are fluid and flexible. "Speed-bumps" along the way may redirect or revise plans.

PAR is a wonderful tool to develop organizational change, to improve nursing practice, or to apply solutions to community concerns because of the active involvement of participants (Stoecker, 2012). Participants in PAR may be part of the decision team at all phases of the project. At the beginning of a project, each participant will have his or her own point of view, but over time, it is expected that these will meld into a new dialogue that reflects a jointly held frame of reference. According to Whyte (1991), the principal investigator (PI) needs to have a good sense of when to contribute and when to refrain from influencing the community of interest. The PI also needs to have a clear understanding of the concepts of power and emancipation so that the desire of the community is inherent to the direction of the study. Mutually agreed upon goals are determined by PI and the participant community.

EXAMPLES OF PAR

Throughout this chapter, I provide examples of my research that used the PAR approach to demonstrate the diversity of PAR applications. Table 3.1 describes each of the projects used as examples.

At the heart of PAR is an ability to follow the community's lead in determining its central concerns (Mohammed et al., 2012). In the AI Proposal, an integral element to the planning grant was the formation of an academic/ tribal team. During the planning period, trust building was an integral part of the goal to explore health disparity from the perspective of the AI (Native American Indian) community. Although the academic team had a very good idea of the major issues confronting the AI community, the PAR method shared power, emancipatory strategies, and collaborative decision making when deciding on priorities in care. Concepts of shared power throughout praxis cannot be overemphasized. In this study, research was proposed with Native Americans; the goal was to form an equitable partnership with our AI community of interest (Schell et al., 2014).

PHILOSOPHICAL RELATIONSHIPS TO PAR

PAR fits within the interpretive research paradigm (Hinchey, 2008). In this milieu, multiple realities are explored with an emphasis on inclusiveness, new ideas, and social construction of knowledge that embrace emancipatory change. These concepts are particularly useful for use with disempowered populations such as AI and other marginalized groups. Kurt Lewin's early theoretical work defines the heart of PAR: reflection and action where the participants are also the researchers (Corbett, Francis, & Chapman, 2007). Lewin believed that there was a symbiotic linkage between problems and issues, and their resolution. In today's world, we might say that those who own the problem need to also own the solutions and have ownership in the process.

Theories such as Lewin's work reflect the concepts of social justice and empowerment and provide a sound theoretical basis for PAR research (Lindsey, Shields, & Stajduhar, 1999). Feminism is another theory that focuses on the marginalization of groups of people who are targets of oppression (Corbett, Francis, & Chapman, 2007). The experience of that oppression is

Table 3.1 *PAR Projects*

Project	Collaborators	Methods	Research Focus/Goal
Planning Network to Improve the Health of New York State Native Americans (AI) (AI Proposal)	Schell and colleagues (2014) and the AI community in a Northeastern region of the United States	Mixed method proposed	Improve health outcomes and reduce disparity in the AI population
Fresh Attitudes: Building Culturally Competent Bridges for Tobacco Control in the Queer Community (Fresh Attitudes)	Bongiorno (2001) and a Northern New England Lesbian, Gay, Bisexual, and Transgender (LGBT) coalition	Qualitative with focus group data collection	Determine the process of building culturally sensitive care in tobacco prevention and control in the LGBT community
Nurses Experiences of the Use of Electronic Health Information Systems in Public Health and Home Care (Nurses EHR)	Bongiorno (2012) and public health nurses in one Northeastern region of the United States	Mixed methods: Quantitative survey and focus groups	Examine nurses' experiences of electronic health information systems in community health
The Experience of Students, Faculty, and Volunteers in a Study Abroad Immersion Experience Focused on Latino Culture, Health and Wellness (Culture and Health)	Bongiorno and Houck (2014) and participants in immersion experience	Ethnography	Explore experience of participants' meanings of own world view, culture, and health
National Study of Quad Council Competencies in Baccalaureate Programs: Survey Results and Recommendations for Practice (Quad Council)	Bongiorno and colleagues (2010) and public health nurses coalition	Quantitative	Identify the practices of baccalaureate granting programs (i.e., BSN) in integrating the Quad Council recommendations in nursing curricula

further segmented by a wide variety of factors such as race, class, ability, nationality, or religion. Feminist theory is committed to examining causes and continuation of oppressive behaviors and works to end oppression. Since PAR emphasizes the decentralization of power as a key construct and feminism examines the centralization of male power in knowledge construction, the use of feminist theory is foundational to PAR research. Feminist theory ensures inclusion of a multitude of voices in the collaborative community of interest, including marginalized voices.

Ethics and Social Justice

The Code of Ethics for Nurses with Interpretive Statements is clear about our responsibility to protect participants in research by assuring them of sufficient information to determine their best course of action (American Nurses Association, 2001). Ethical issues in PAR require considerable care because of the nature of PAR's philosophy. PAR epitomizes the concepts of patient-centered ethical decision trees, which means to work with people rather than do things to people. This partnership in action can create some difficulties with informed consent or voluntary withdrawal. If the research is being conducted in a small setting, participants may feel the need to be accepted by the group and its norms, making it difficult to decline to participate or to later withdraw. Once an individual agrees to participate, due to the group nature of the work, the individual may find it difficult to withdraw as he or she may not want to disappoint the group. When conducting research in a small group setting, allowing for privacy to enroll or withdraw is an important consideration.

Social justice is a commitment that is ingrained in the design and execution of PAR studies. The complexity of social justice within an ethnic context can pose many challenges for research groups because of disparity and power inequalities (Johnston-Goldstar, 2013). Health disparity is greatest among AI, African American, Hispanic, and lesbian, gay, bisexual, and transgender (LGBT) communities. These are also groups who have often been victimized. Marginalized groups may struggle to trust researchers when those researchers belong to an ethnic group whose historical, collective actions have done untold harm (Adams et al., 2013). When working with oppressed groups, it is vital to integrate acknowledgment of previous wrongs into the trust building process.

Measures to ensure informed consent are most important (Lofman, Pelkonen, & Pietila, 2004). Research studies should be approved by the institutional review board (IRB). Use of the IRB application ensures protection for the participants, including that the study will be led by qualified persons. It should also discuss the approach to any special care needs of vulnerable groups.

In the Culture and Health study, all group members were required to participate in the same activities for course credit, whether they enrolled in the study or not. Privacy was afforded to all participants to enroll. These measures ensured that the small group experience was comfortable for all, regardless of status as a participant in the research (Bongiorno & Houck, 2014). In the Nurses Electronic Health Record (EHR) study, privacy was ensured by enrollment by mail or by separate discussion prior to survey completion and focus group discussion at regional workshops (Bongiorno, 2012).

PRACTICAL VALUE OF PAR

One of the joys of PAR is that it generally leads to action. Awareness is raised about an issue, and the process of PAR lays down a foundation for change. According to Corbett and colleagues (2007), to obtain results, a group needs to perform three actions: determine the nature of the issue to be explored, gather participants, and operationalize the results into action.

The Culture and Health project demonstrates the usefulness of PAR (Bongiorno & Houck, 2014). A like-minded group shared a common sense of awareness of a lack of opportunity in the curriculum to explore cultural competency. The reflective work led to development of an immersion program in Mexico. During the immersion, participants in the program were able to co-examine their own cycle of socialization and discuss their ingrained cultural values in relation to experiences in host communities. Participants also explored host country cultural, family, and community norms and used photo journaling and storytelling as ways to examine their underlying values. Course corrections throughout the immersion added new depth and ideas to the focus of research. As a result of the PAR approach, participants shared a new understanding of the context of diversity awareness and cultural competency in health and wellness. In the final action phase, participants collaborated to discuss findings and integrated meanings of cultural competency in health and wellness.

BACKGROUND AND COLLABORATIVE DIALOGUE

PAR begins with a collaborative dialogue among the PI and the group of interest during which they define the area of interest and discuss underlying group values. Groups consider issues where an exploration might lead to ideas for change. The conceptual phase should build in enough time to achieve trust and engagement by the participants.

Collaborative dialogue is a vital step where groups sort through multiple ideas, organize a cohesive focus, and develop mutually agreeable procedures for the research to move forward (Whyte, 1991). The process might include an advisory board or a steering committee or simply be a group of participants and the primary researcher conjoined in the quest for answers to a problem. The nature of the partnership varies widely from one where community members are involved in every part of the process to structures where there is a less equal allocation of power (D'Alonzo, 2010). Here we offer several examples of ways to establish the background for a study.

The Nurses EHR study began with discussions of "rollout" issues in public health departments where nurses were transitioning from paper to electronic documentation systems (Bongiorno, 2012). Nurses were experiencing great distress over the transition and voiced a lack of understanding of the benefits of a new system. The group had many questions, chief among which were concerns about the nature of transition and the relationship between quality and safety and use of EHR. The process from concept to data collection was months in the making.

Another example relates the power of collaborative dialogue. A group of public health educators and supervisors in the field discussed widely varying preparation of nurses in public health, which created major issues in hiring and orientation practices. The Quad Council studies were born out of the group's reflection on these issues (Bongiorno et al., 2010; Mullarkey et al., 2009). The group worked together for several years to complete the task of answering the community's concerns.

The AI Proposal began with concern over a lack of access to care and health disparity among AI populations. Further exploration by a diverse group of academics led to a proposal for a planning grant, whose aim was to develop trust and explore disparity with the AI community. The goal was to build a strong relationship that could tackle health issues of interest, ones driven by the needs and desires of the AI community (Schell et al., 2014). In this work, the proposal included the AI community at the very start of the project to gain buy-in, despite the awareness that developing a partnership of equality would be a time-consuming process, taking at least a year before actual work on research could ensue.

REVIEWING THE LITERATURE

A review of the literature shares what is known about the area of inquiry and considers previous approaches to concerns. Exploring the state of the science of phenomena helps to determine the focus of research questions and guides development of new knowledge (Polit & Beck, 2014). A solid literature review tells a story of strengths and gaps in knowledge about the topic that creates a framework for understanding by the researcher. The literature review may be likened to solving a picture puzzle: All of the pieces are related, but it is up to the person trying to solve the puzzle to develop relationships that make sense. If a puzzle piece is missing, it becomes quite clear as construction comes to a close. This is how synthesis of the literature is a key element (Houser, 2012). Review of the literature may occur before or after data collection and data analysis, depending on the research design.

For example, in the Fresh Attitudes study, concerns ran high as to why tobacco use rates were high in the LGBT community (Bongiorno, 2001). Because the PAR group was not well versed in tobacco prevention specific to the LGBT community, a preresearch literature review was vitally important in establishing baseline data. It became quickly apparent that each of the communities within the LGBT umbrella had unique needs and stressors, so the original plan to partner with all of these groups was reframed to focus on each of the distinct groups as separate research studies. The literature review also synthesized ideas on how to approach the LGBT communities and gain trust. Synthesis of results empowered the group's co-direction of the study and helped to determine the strengths and gaps in knowledge about the research.

DEVELOPMENT OF THE RESEARCH QUESTION

The development of the research question often includes both the PI and the participants in the research. Often, the research question comes from the participants' experiences within the community of interest (Stoecker, 2012). Some studies use an immersion approach to examine phenomena of interest while developing the research questions. Immersion also encourages extensive dialogue and intensive engagement in the process (Gregg et al., 2013).

An example of the intimate nature of immersion, as it relates to development of the research question, is seen in the Culture and Health study, where participants spent 3 weeks immersed in the rural indigenous culture of Mexico. The group started out with wide variation in conceptual thinking but gradually bracketed preconceptions to form a more holistic awareness of the meaning of the experience (Bongiorno & Houck, 2014). The development of the research questions for Fresh Attitudes was less intensive but was determined by a team of key informants from the LGBT community (Bongiorno, 2001). The group sifted through many ideas to conclude with a specific aim to examine perceptions of smoking and to explore underlying causes of smoking in the community. They considered how answers to these questions might inform health promotion changes in the community. Many additional questions were also considered as the research focus took shape.

SIGNIFICANCE

In framing research questions, the PI needs to consider significance. Because PAR is about using research to translate into action, the consequences of the research have to be considered (Izumi et al., 2010). In the Fresh Attitudes study, the direction of the research questions was influenced by the group's desire to include policy level change and patient advocacy. In the other examples in this chapter, each potential outcome or change was related to a meritorious concern and one that would lead to community or education change for a more equitable health state among patients.

SCIENTIFIC RIGOR

PAR is a scientifically rigorous approach to research using constructivist ideals. This approach is generally concerned more with reliability than validity, because studies are often local and with fewer participants (Williamson, Bellman, & Webster, 2012). The reflexive nature of PAR incorporates action, reflection, and action (ARA) cycles. This dynamic process has been criticized because of the subjective insertion of situational factors as the research progresses. The proximity of the researcher to the PAR process also generates criticism. Counterarguments share that rigor can be interpreted as the disclosure of the process in PAR, a strength that crystalizes validity through the ARA cycle.

In the Tacit Dimension, Polanyi (1966) says in his historical analysis of tacit knowledge that *we know more than we can say*. His treatise lends great credibility to the scientific rigor of the PAR approach because its credence lies in engaging the tacit knowledge of a group to form an explicit analysis of problem-based change. Scientific rigor is further strengthened in PAR by using strategies such as triangulation, confirming accuracy of findings with participants, and consulting expert panels to validate data. The bottom line is that regardless of critics, PAR focuses on new knowledge acquisition using established research methods within an emancipatory approach. Scientific rigor is inherent in this process.

METHODS

Research Design

The key feature in a design that uses a PAR approach is to embed community participation (Mubuuke & Leibowitz, 2013). The design is a guide for the researcher, driven by the research questions, to build convincing evidence that answers the research question (Hinchey, 2008). Design is a logical process from which flows sampling, setting, and procedures and includes the basic principles of inquiry. Teasing out the differences between causation and correlation or prediction is an important factor in considering design (Rebar, Gersch, Macnee, & McCabe, 2011). The research design determines the process of examining a problem, developing questions, organizing methods, and determining analysis, conclusions, and dissemination (Creswell, 2007). The careful application of design principles to PAR research is a fundamental principle when determining validity of results. It is the blueprint used to develop a comprehensive work plan.

The examples of research cited earlier in this chapter all used the PAR approach with a variety of research designs. In each case, the participants brainstormed problems, methods of inquiry, and possible actions that might result. The design process may take time because the PAR approach is inclusive. The PI often co-engages in the work with a good number of team members who have little working knowledge of the research process and may have educational and other challenges to consider (Ganann, 2013). In a community problem-solving process, honoring the contribution of all partners is essential to success. The engagement of stakeholders requires patience, tact, and purposeful planning. Efforts are well rewarded as the perspectives of the community are integrated into the research design.

Work Plan

The work plan is the "to do" list, which includes projected timelines. It incorporates elements of the overall research process, such as considering ideas for developing instruments and evaluation procedures. The work plan also includes the more mundane aspects of the project like organizing meeting dates, establishing guidelines for communication, and ordering supplies. It is also a good idea for a work plan to establish and link goals, objectives, activities, and outcomes. The complexity of the work plan depends on the nature and scope of the study or project (Chevalier & Buckles, 2011).

Research Cycle

In PAR, each step of the design process or research cycle can potentially integrate change into an organization, thus becoming an action cycle (Whyte, 1991). The cyclical nature is shown in this example. *Reflection:* In the Culture and Health project, the research team was concerned with professional students' lack of ability to internalize the core concepts of diversity awareness into cultural competency with marginalized populations (Bongiorno & Houck, 2014). The curriculum clearly exhibited a gap in operationalizing concepts of diversity awareness. This led to considering ways to improve their awareness of how and why worldviews develop, evolve, and influence care. *Action:* A research question was developed: Would immersion in a semester- long study-abroad program in nursing improve students' ability to reflect on their own worldview? The problem identification and gap in education linked reflection and action to a research hypothesis: Students who engage in a study-abroad immersion program will improve their understanding of how their worldview impacts cultural competence in practice. The sample would consist of professional students in the sophomore through senior years. This action was a change in curriculum. *Reflection:* Results from this study are ongoing, with participants vigorous in keeping datasets and sharing learning through focus groups and other methods. *Action:* On an annual basis, the group has disseminated process evaluations that have deepened understanding among faculty and administration, thereby institutionalizing the concepts and diffusing change. As seen in Figure 3.1, the cycle from the Fresh Attitudes study explains the nature of action and reflection as a symbiotic circle of knowledge acquisition and application.

As the action design is planned, it is important to assess the research question(s) and purpose to help the investigative team decide on a research method. For example, to compare an intervention effect one would design a randomized controlled trial, but if one wanted to know how to explore meanings or lifeways, a qualitative method would be the more appropriate choice (Kneipp et al., 2011). The important concept to remember in the design process is that the outcome of the work should answer the research question,

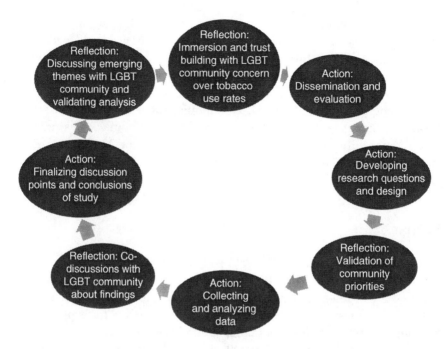

Figure 3.1 *Example of PAR cycle of reflection and action with Fresh Attitudes study.*

help to close the gap between theory and practice, and provide useful solutions to a problem (Jaqosh et al., 2012). The structure of the design is seldom linear but is recursive, where new knowledge leads the researchers to review previously held ideas (Williamson, Bellman, & Webster, 2012). Emerging data or themes will inform the design as it moves forward. PAR design is flexible, dynamic, and emancipatory—a journey.

Sample

Sampling methods are driven by the research questions and design. Because PAR is inclusive, the questions would generally be prioritized from the perspective of the research partners and be purposive. This is not a linear process; changes or additions to focus may occur through the inquiry as new information emerges (Munhall, 2007). The importance of sampling procedures in a qualitative study is to select participants who have experience with the phenomena of interest. For quantitative projects, it is equally important to be sure the sample also matches the population of interest. The goal of a quality sampling plan is always to avoid bias in the sample, which leads to distorted results (Polit & Beck, 2014).

For example, in Fresh Attitudes, the sample was one of convenience but limited to those who self-identified as being within the LGBT sexual orientation (Bongiorno, 2001). Each subset of inquiry further stratified the sample parameters by age group and gender identification. In some PAR studies, an entire community would be part of the sample, as in the AI Proposal. Every member of the AI nations in one Northeastern location was an eligible study participant, although perhaps with different degrees of involvement.

Setting

The setting for action research might be better characterized as the context of inquiry. Because topics of study cover a range of subjects and can use a wide variety of research methods, consider the community of interest as the setting. Action research is often carried out in classrooms for exploration of teaching/learning strategies or implementation of a new initiative such as in the Culture and Health initiative. Other times the community of interest is on a national level, and a core group of participants guide much of the study, as in the Quad Council study. One setting in the Fresh Attitudes study was at a gay pride parade festival, where gay men were interviewed on location.

Instruments and Data Collection

The use of data collection methods varies widely. The important consideration is to determine if the instrument provides quality information to answer the research questions. In the Quad Council study, the group decided on a pilot study to lend greater validity to the instrument to be used in future work. Triangulated methods were best suited to the Nurses EMR study, using a written survey and focus group interviews, to provide a broad cross-section of data. Fresh Attitudes used qualitative instruments, such as focus groups and interviews, as these were best suited to the level of context needed in the design. The Culture and Health study questions also were best answered with the richness of experience that is inherent in instruments such as journals, interviews, and focus groups.

There are advantages and disadvantages in each method of data collection (Polit & Beck, 2014). Surveys may use questions that are biased, response rates may be low, and respondents may answer what they think the researcher wants to hear. Conversely, surveys provide easy acquisition of demographic information and are an appropriate tool to measure objective information with large numbers of people. Qualitative methods are more time consuming and may not be suitable for some vulnerable populations. Focus groups are often recorded, which can make some participants uneasy or unwilling to share information. The quality of recordings also sometimes loses important contextual data. Nevertheless, qualitative data provide a richness and context that cannot be elicited by quantitative methods. Reflective field journals and photo journals personalize meanings and can build case studies or add to other methods used in a study.

Data Analysis

Data analysis is directly related to the research design. In PAR, data analysis might be shared by the group or led by the PI but with some level of group interpretation. The members of the research study should validate the results (Whyte, 1991). In the Quad Council study, interested participants were sent the results of the study for comment (Bongiorno et al., 2010). In Fresh Attitudes, the group met together and discussed all of the outcomes (Bongiorno, 2001). The AI Proposal also included procedures for validation in the plan (Schell et al., 2014).

Findings

The work plan can be a helpful tool in crafting the findings report. The records may prompt the PI to discuss the cyclical process of the study and how it influenced data collection. As in any study, the datasets need to be fully explored, and qualitative findings examined for meaning. For example, the Nurses EHR preliminary findings were discussed among interested participants at a wide variety of meetings, prompting a revision of the survey for future inquiry (Bongiorno, 2012).

Discussion

The culmination of a PAR study lies in its discussion and subsequent dissemination. This is the place to examine findings and consider how they answered research question(s). The discussion should analyze how the study results fill the theory/practice gap or strengthen the threads of current knowledge in the field. It is important to discuss key points, such as problems in the research, failures, as well as major findings. Also, make sure the discussion adds new knowledge, discusses limitations, and considers lessons learned. Fresh Attitudes linked feminist theory to why smoking rates were high (Bongiorno, 2001). A major theme found throughout that body of work was disparity in stress levels and a heightened sense of cognitive dissonance in the LGBT study community. The research group concluded that, for prevention and cessation of tobacco use in the population, they needed to focus on these two concepts as central to health promotion efforts.

Conclusion

This chapter discussed the basic strategies and theoretical underpinnings of PAR. Multiple examples explored the application of the PAR approach to research. The conclusion section of a PAR study should be short and recap the primary focus of the topic. Recommendations for future work should also be discussed. Final thoughts on the study, such as words of wisdom, can be added, including how findings are relevant to practice and lessons learned.

REFERENCES

Adams, M., Blumenfeld, W., Castenada, C., Hackman, H., Peters, M., & Zuniga, X. (Eds.). (2013). *Readings for diversity and social justice* (3rd ed.). New York, NY: Routledge.

American Nurses Association. (2001). *Code of ethics for nurses with interpretive statements.* Silver Spring, MD: American Nurses Publishing.

Bongiorno, A. (2001, November). *Fresh attitudes in increasing diversity/eliminating disparities: Understanding and implementing concepts.* Paper presented at the National Conference on Tobacco or Health. New Orleans, LA.

Bongiorno, A. (2012, March). *EHR: Electronic health records for community nursing.* Paper presented at New York State Teachers Union Professional Issues Forum on Health Care. Albany, NY.

Bongiorno, A., & Houck, N. (2014). *The experience of students, faculty, and volunteers in a study abroad immersion experience focused on Latino culture, health and wellness.* Unpublished manuscript.

Bongiorno, A., Mullarkey, M., Clemmens, D., Fletcher, M., Riegle, B., & Nelson, N. (2010, November). *National survey results: Comparing Quad Council competencies to preparation of nurses in baccalaureate nursing programs.* Presented at the American Public Health Association Annual International Meeting. Washington, DC.

Chevalier, J., & Buckles, D. (2011). *A handbook for participatory action research, planning and evaluation.* Retrieved from http://www.participatoryactionresearch.net/sites/default/files/sites/all/files/manager/pdf/sas2_module1_sept11_red_en.pdf

Corbett, M., Francis, K., & Chapman, Y. (2007). Feminist-informed participatory action research: A methodology of choice for examining critical nursing issues. *International Journal of Nursing Practice, 13,* 81–88.

Creswell, J. (2007). *Qualitative inquiry and research design choosing among five approaches.* (2nd ed.). Thousand Oaks, CA: Sage Publications.

D'Alonzo, K. (2010). Getting started in CBPR: Lessons in building community partnerships for new researchers. *Nursing Inquiry, 17*(4), 282–288.

Ganann, R. (2013). Opportunities and challenges associated with engaging immigrant women in participatory action research. *Journal of Immigrant Minority Health, 15,* 341–349.

Gregg, K., Irwin, R., Houck, N. M., Zoucha, R., Stayer, D., Kattan, B., . . . Turk, M. (2013). Fieldwork as a way of knowing: An Italian immersion experience. *Online Journal of Cultural Competence in Nursing and Healthcare, 3*(3), 16–30. doi:10.9730/ojccnh.org/v3n3a2

Hinchey, P. (2008). *Action research.* New York, NY: Peter Lang.

Houser, J. (2012). Nursing research reading, using and creating evidence (2nd ed.). Sudbury, MA: Jones & Bartlett.

Izumi, B., Schulz, A., Israel, B., Reyes, A., Martin, J., Lichtenstein, R., . . . Sand, S. (2010). The one-pager: A practical advocacy tool for translating community-based participatory research into action. *Progress in Community Health Partnerships, 4*(2), 141–147.

Jaqosh, J., MacCaulay, A., Pluye, P., Salsberg, J., Bush, P., Henderson, J., . . . Greenhalgh, T. (2012). Uncovering the benefits of participatory research: Implications for a realist review for health research and practice. *Milbank Quarterly, 90*(2), 311–317.

Johnston-Goodstar, K. (2013). Indigenous youth participatory action research: Re-visioning social justice for social work with Indigenous youths. *Social Work, 58*(4), 314–320.

Kneipp, S., Kairalla, J., Lutz, B., Pereira, D., Hall, A., Flocks, J., . . . Schwartz, T. (2011). Public health nursing case management for women receiving temporary assistance for needy families: A randomized controlled trial using community-based participatory research. *American Journal of Public Health, 101*(9), 1759–1768.

Lindsey, E., Shields, L., & Stajduhar, K. (1999). Creating effective nursing partnerships: Relating community development to participatory action research. *Journal of Advanced Nursing, 29*(5), 1238–1245.

Lofman, P., Pelkonen, M., & Pietila, A. M. (2004). Ethical issues in participatory action research. *Scandinavian Journal of Caring Science, 18*(3), 333–340.

Mohammed, S., Walters, K., LaMarr, J., Evans-Campbell, T., & Fryberg, S. (2012). Finding middle ground: Negotiating university and tribal community interests in community-based participatory action research. *Nursing Inquiry, 19*(2), 116–127. doi:10.1111/j.1440-1800.2011.00557.x

Mubuuke, A. G., & Leibowitz, B. (2013). Participatory action research: The key to successful implementation of innovations in health professions education. *African Journal of Health Professions Education, 5*(1), 30–33.

Mullarkey, M., Bongiorno, A., Clemmens, D., Fletcher, M., Riegle, B., & Nelson, N. (2009, November). *Comparing Quad Council competencies to preparation of nurses in baccalaureate nursing programs. Pilot.* Presented at the American Public Health Association Annual International Meeting. Washington, DC.

Munhall, P. (2007). *Nursing research: A qualitative perspective* (4th ed.). Sudbury, MA: Jones & Bartlett.

Polanyi, M. (1966). *The tacit dimension.* New York, NY: Doubleday & Company.

Polit, D., & Beck, C. (2014). *Essentials of nursing research appraising evidence for nursing practice* (8th ed.). Philadelphia, PA: Wolters Kluwer Lippincott Williams & Wilkins.

Rebar, C., Gersch, C., Macnee, C., & McCabe, S. (2011). *Understanding nursing research in evidence-based practice* (3rd ed.). Philadelphia, PA: Wolters Kluwer/Lippincott Williams & Wilkins.

Schell, L. B., Bongiorno, A. W., Bonner, K., Hodges, B., DiVita, M., & Peabody, C. (2014). *Planning network to improve health of New York's Native Americans.* Unpublished Research Proposal Manuscript. Albany, NY: State University of New York.

Simonds, V., & Christopher, S. (2013). Adapting Western research methods to Indigenous ways of knowing. *American Journal of Public Health, 103*(12), 2185–2192.

Stoecker, R. (2012). *Research methods for community change a project based approach* (2nd ed.). Thousand Oaks, CA: Sage.

Whyte, W. (1991). *Participatory action research.* Newbury Park, CA: Sage.

Williamson, G., Bellman, L., & Webster, J. (2012). *Action research in nursing and healthcare.* Los Angeles, CA: Sage Publications.

CHAPTER FOUR

AN ASSESSMENT OF A PROTOTYPE AUDIT AND FEEDBACK PROCESS TO IMPROVE INPATIENT PAIN DOCUMENTATION

Matthew Peters

*T*his chapter is an abstracted sample of a participatory action research (PAR) proposal and represents the actual dissertation of the author. Because the study is in progress and because dissertations cannot be reprinted in full in a volume such as this, the author has selected key aspects of the design to discuss and included the following commentary by the author's dissertation chair.

THE STUDY

This dissertation reports on a PAR study that will use an automated process to abstract and report feedback on nurses' previous pain documentation within an inpatient nursing unit. The clinical data will come from an electronic medical record (EMR), where the data abstraction is automated via an enterprise data warehouse (EDW). The EDW aggregates the data, and the results will be organized in a series of research iterations into a final version of a feedback report that the nurse can view on an intranet.

The basis for the research comes from the existing literature on clinician audit and feedback, one definition of which is "any summary of clinical performance of health care over a specified period of time, given in a written, electronic or verbal format" (Jamtvedt, Young, Kristoffersen, O'Brien, & Oxman, 2006, p. 102). Audit and feedback is also known as performance feedback. For this study, audit and feedback is defined as a process that audits a nurse's previous clinical documentation to give information back to the nurse to maintain or improve documentation.

My academic interest in nurse audit and feedback and my full-time work as a nurse informaticist have always influenced each other. Early in my career as a nurse manager, I was amazed at the amount of time and effort inpatient nursing units put into manual audit and feedback, with little impact on patient outcomes. I was surprised at how much clinician documentation on patient care was entered into an EMR with no options for easy retrieval. The only way to measure the efficacy of care was with tremendous manual effort to collate feedback from the EMR. As I subsequently focused on and learned about abstracting data electronically from EMRs, I gained an appreciation for the complexity of such a task. But once all work has been completed in automating electronic data abstraction and redisplaying it for feedback, the benefit is reaped by giving all clinicians access to information about their clinical care and its effects on patient outcomes. Once clinicians learn how their care may vary from best practices, they are able to make changes that could dramatically improve thousands of patients' lives (Archibald et al., 2011). When done correctly, audit and feedback is very effective; what is missing in current research is a definition of the most effective way to do it.

Improving Patient Outcomes

Motivations

Within our national health care system, there has been continuing emphasis on decreasing patient harm and improving health care quality (Kohn, Corrigan, & Donaldson, 2000; Kohn, Corrigan, & Donaldson, 2001, p. 1). Hospitals have come to realize that they must improve quality of care or they will lose money. To incentivize quality care in hospitals, the Centers for Medicare and Medicaid (CMS) have introduced pay-for-performance initiatives over the last 5 years. In October 2007, the CMS implemented payment rule CMS-1533-FC, which stops payment to hospitals for hospital-acquired conditions. As of October 2012, performance on CMS value-based purchasing (VBP) measures is now tied to financial penalties. If a hospital does not meet the VBP performance standard, CMS will hold back a percentage of the hospital's payments for services. For example, the Illinois Hospital Association predicted that its hospitals would lose $41 million from VBP in reimbursement based on its overall performance in 2007, with a 1% penalty in fiscal year 2013 (Illinois Hospital Association, 2011). Thus, the motivation to improve performance has financial implications. Audit and feedback, which has already been used to improve the quality of health care, could also potentially be used to meet these pay-for-performance initiatives.

Cochrane Review

In 2006, Jamtvedt, Young, Kristoffersen, O'Brien, and Oxman performed a Cochrane Review on audit and feedback, reviewing 118 research studies involving physicians and/or their practices. The authors concluded that "it is striking how little can be discerned about the effects of audit and feedback based on the 118 trials included in this review" (2006, p. 22). The review demonstrated that much remains to be understood about clinician performance feedback. The analysis used only quantitative, randomized control trials. Although not a measured outcome, the Cochrane Review proposed that one factor in predicting whether audit and feedback would be effective was whether the health care professional's participation in the study was active or passive. In other words, the more active the health care professional was in the overall audit and feedback process and the more responsible he or she was for implementing changes, the more effective would be the audit and feedback.

Nurses at the Center of Change

Nurses are the largest group of health care professionals in the United States and play a critical role in efforts to improve health care (Committee on the Robert Wood Johnson Foundation Initiative on the Future of Nursing, 2011; Hughes, 2008). Logically, those who provide care must be involved in the process to improve it. The Robert Wood Johnson initiative of transforming care at the bedside (TCAB) has shown that when frontline nurses are actively involved in efforts to improve health care, the results are very effective (Needleman et al., 2007). This, in addition to the results of the Cochrane Review on audit and feedback noted earlier (Jamtvedt et al., 2006), shows the importance of including frontline clinicians in developing feedback.

Collecting and Evaluating Data

At the same time, the data collected and used for the audit and feedback process are just as critical. An evaluation of TCAB showed that 83% of nurse managers thought that collecting and analyzing data was the most important task of all 23 TCAB activities; 31% also rated it as one of the most difficult (Parkerton et al., 2009). In addition, of all barriers encountered in the TCAB process, insufficient staff time to participate in TCAB was rated the highest (Parkerton et al., 2009). In other words, nurses understand the importance of collecting data and recognize it as their most challenging task, yet limits on their available time restrict their participation in these projects. Data collection, analysis, and time to participate are thus all barriers in the audit and feedback process.

After the Department of Veterans Affairs observed in 1985 that postoperative morbidity and mortality were high in the Veterans Affairs (VA) Health System, Congress mandated that the VA periodically benchmark its postoperative outcomes to those of the private sector (Ingraham, Richards, Hall, & Ko, 2010). Eventually this led to the creation of the National Surgical Quality Improvement Project (NSQIP), run by the American College of Surgeons. The NSQIP program allows hospitals to submit data on surgical cases and, in return, receive benchmark scores on how well they have performed on various risk-adjusted outcomes compared with other participating hospitals. The program has demonstrated significant improvements in 30-day postoperative morbidity and mortality in both VA and private sector hospitals (Ingraham et al., 2010).

Collecting and analyzing reliable data lies at the foundation of the NSQIP and its success. All data submitted to the NSQIP are manually abstracted by clinical nurse reviewers. According to Hammermeister (2009):

> This model was essential to the NSQIP's initial success in the era of the handwritten medical record. … It has become clear to me that the cost of the current method of data collection has become the Achilles' heel of the NSQIP. (p. S69)

The strength of having clinical nurse reviewers abstract the data manually lies in the quality of data submitted to NSQIP. A limiting factor in manually abstracting data, however, is the slow, methodical process needed to perform the abstraction, requiring an expensive clinical nurse reviewer. Only so much data can be submitted to NSQIP by a single clinical nurse reviewer, thus limiting the collection of data to a surgical specialty (e.g., general surgery, vascular surgery) rather than the population of all surgical specialties. But increased use of EMRs and the ability to automate the abstraction of data into an EDW could eliminate the need for manual audits and initiate the move to semiautomated audits, allowing data abstraction to be extended to other surgical specialty areas and freeing up nurses' time from collecting data to focusing on improving health care.

Enterprise Data Warehousing and Data Analysis

Health care systems use hundreds of different computer programs to run their business and document care of their patients. Most data on these computer programs are stored on differently designed databases that do not communicate with one another. To stay viable and improve patient outcomes, health care systems need to combine all data into a single database. This idea is similar to bringing together all the nations of the world into a single location (such as the United Nations in New York), providing a setting where everyone can dialogue with one another (via interpreters) to solve the world's problems. Likewise, a health care EDW abstracts data from different computer programs, such as the lab, radiology, finance, pharmacy, transfusion services, and EMR systems, and combines them into a single database to be analyzed.

One current strategy for limiting the labor in manual audit and feedback is to sample a representation of the overall population. This method of measurement, however, is limited to the representativeness of the chosen population sample. Also, some health care quality issues, such as collaterally acquired conditions associated with an inpatient hospital stay, may be mismeasured owing to the sampling technique. These conditions include ventilator-assisted pneumonia, catheter-associated urinary tract infections (CAUTI), central line-associated bloodstream infections, deep venous thrombosis, and pressure ulcers. The protocols for preventing these from occurring are well established but poorly audited. Because acquiring one of these conditions is not common, the performance goal may be to reduce the rate of CAUTIs from 2 in 1,000 patient days to 1 in 10,000. The EDW's ability to automate data collection on all patient data would eliminate the need for sampling and could create better quality feedback in preventing these hospital-acquired conditions.

Other health care performance problems involve patient safety. These are typically more common problems related to failing to follow an established treatment protocol. Some examples of patient safety issues include falls, medication errors, patient injury, and so forth. Failure to follow the established protocol does not mean that a patient will be harmed, but it does increase the likelihood of harm. Manual audit and feedback creates a time delay between delivering actual care and giving feedback to clinicians, thus propagating potential patient safety events. Audit and feedback supported by an EDW, on the other hand, would increase the proximity of the feedback to the time the care occurred. Having timely feedback regarding compliance with patient safety protocols would permit better monitoring and the taking of action if necessary.

One measurement within VBP is the Hospital Consumer Assessment of Healthcare Providers and Systems (HCAHPS). This is a survey given to patients after discharge from the hospital about the perceptions of the care they received. As hospitals try to improve performance on the HCAHPS survey, many of the interventions implemented to meet these goals are being documented in the EMR (e.g., rounding on patients hourly, updating goals on a white board, giving out educational handouts). But because EMR data are stored in a different database from the results of the HCAHPS data, it becomes difficult to compare both datasets to see if the interventions have made a difference in improving HCAHPS scores. A main function of the EDW would be to aggregate data from disparate databases into a single source for analysis, and so this barrier would be easily overcome. Being able to compare data from disparate databases in one report increases the data's value to clinicians, and the data are more likely to influence change if needed.

Learning Environment

Yet even with excellent data for clinicians to review, the environment of the inpatient nursing unit may still pose barriers to improving patient outcomes. One question is whether this environment actually supports "learning from failure." Drach-Zahavy and Pud (2010) evaluated the learning environments of 32 surgical and internal wards and showed that only 13% had environments conducive to learning from failures. Tucker and Edmondson (2003) described how using highly skilled individual clinicians to prevent medical errors in health care, as done previously, was no longer a viable solution and suggested that preventing medical errors in the future would be solved by better organization and management. As summarized in the literature, a learning environment consists of collecting and analyzing data, drawing conclusions, implementing changes, and having an integrated process whereby all frontline clinicians are involved in the process (Drach-Zahavy & Pud, 2010; Tucker & Edmondson, 2003). For example, instead of having a nurse from the quality department perform chart audits and return the results to the nurse manager for improvement, the inpatient unit nurses would participate in the audits, analyze the results, come to a conclusion, and implement the change. Having nurses involved in the entire process is known as an integrated approach, as opposed to a nonintegrated approach that uses nurses who are not on the front line. Thus, creating a learning environment is a prerequisite for feedback to be effective.

PROBLEM STATEMENT

With mounting financial risk, hospitals need to improve patient outcomes. Yet despite hundreds of research studies on audit and feedback, little is understood about its efficacy. To that end I have identified five factors that affect the effectiveness of audit and feedback. First, the literature on clinical process improvement, which typically includes audit and feedback, has shown that integrating frontline nurses into the overall process improves patient outcomes (Jamtvedt et al., 2006; Needleman, Kurtzman, & Kizer, 2007). Second, although collecting and analyzing data is a key component in this process, existing manual methods mitigate its benefit. Third, automating the collection and audit of data via an EDW and making the feedback available on an intranet could improve audit and feedback. Fourth, an integrated learning environment contributes to the overall process. Finally, feedback needs to be based on a proven theoretical model for changing behavior, an issue that provides a starting point for this study.

To examine and analyze these factors, a manual audit and feedback process, that is, a medical record review (MDR), will be compared to an automated audit and feedback process using an EDW to create the feedback. The setting for this study will be in a medical–surgical unit at a community hospital. The topic for this audit and feedback comparison will be compliance to charting of three different pain assessments as required by the hospital protocol. The participatory action component of the study involves frontline nurses in successive cycles of feedback specification.

This study therefore seeks to implement a collaborative, nurse-centered process for providing feedback on pain documentation performance, as guided by Bandura's (1991) social cognitive theory of self-regulation. To that end, it will use an EDW to assemble the audit data and a feedback process developed with nurse participation. Findings will help assess the potential for future replications of this feedback approach and design in other care arenas. The long-term goal of this program of research on care processes is to harness the power of an EDW to create performance feedback, thereby humanizing the engagement of nurses in providing optimal care to patients.

STUDY AIMS AND RESEARCH QUESTIONS

For any comparison study, a baseline must be established. The first aim of this study is to understand nurses' perceptions of the purpose, benefits, and drawbacks of the current MDR audit and feedback process. This involves establishing their general overall knowledge of the two audit and feedback processes (MDR and EDW prototype). The nurses will be asked research questions 1 and 2 at the beginning of the study for the MDR process and again at the end of the study for the EDW prototype process.

1. Research question 1: According to nurses, what is the purpose of the audit and feedback process?
2. Research question 2: What do nurses perceive to be the benefits and drawbacks of the audit and feedback process?

The second aim of this study is to develop and describe a prototype process, based on Bandura's (1991) social cognitive theory of self-regulation, for using the EDW to create an automated audit and feedback report for pain management protocols in a collaborative and participatory setting with frontline nurses, and then analyze what was learned throughout the process. Research questions 3 and 4 address these issues:

3. Research question 3: What was collaboratively learned in creating audit and feedback with frontline nurses that would improve the future development of this prototype?
4. Research question 4: What changes (format, content, delivery) need to be made from the initial to final version of the feedback and why?

The final aim focuses on comparing and contrasting the peer-reviewed MDR and the collaborative automated EDW process for creating audit and feedback with respect to documentation outcomes and nurses' preferences, if any. Research questions 5 and 6 deal with these issues:

5. Research question 5: Does charting compliance with pain assessments (Table 4.1) improve using the sequential versions of the audit and feedback prototype process?
6. Research question 6: What do nurses think about the relative merits, if any, in using the prototype audit and feedback process over the peer-reviewed MDR process?

SIGNIFICANCE

This study complements work already done with TCAB by developing performance feedback with frontline nurses, using a participatory approach that explores ways to use electronic nursing documentation to improve nursing documentation. Using an EDW to develop nurse performance feedback has many inherent benefits that may overcome many of the existing barriers in developing and delivering feedback and making it more meaningful. This research could thus lead to a paradigm shift in how feedback on nursing performance is developed.

Methods

Central to this study is a methodology that focuses on progressive cycles of assessing and improving performance feedback that is driven by frontline clinicians and what they value. One such methodology is PAR. The strength of PAR lies in its ability to empower and engage those receiving performance feedback to use and improve it (Meyer, 2000). Herr and Anderson (2005, p. 5) have described the cyclical nature of PAR: "This cycle of activities forms an action research spiral in which each cycle increases the researchers' knowledge of the original question, puzzle, or problem and, it is hoped, leads to its solution" (p. 5). The key statement in this quotation is "increases the researchers' knowledge," emphasizing the importance of the learning that takes place during this process. Concerning value, Herr and Anderson observed that, "like all forms of inquiry, action research is *value laden*" (2005, p. 4). In other words, if the researchers do not value the research or its expected outcome, little or no change will occur in an action research study. It is unrealistic to expect that doing a single assessment and intervention would create valid knowledge. Instead, knowledge is developed slowly over time by performing multiple cycles of planning, acting, observing, and reflecting.

Overview of Study

The remainder of the dissertation will be developed as follows. First, an in-depth overview of the motivators to improve patient outcomes is provided, followed by a review of the application of theory to improve audit and feedback in health care processes such as documentation of pain management. This is followed by highlights of the PAR methodology and the overall design for this study. Then the summary of what was learned in creating audit and feedback using an EDW to provide nurses' feedback, designed according to Bandura's self-regulation theory, is presented. Finally, as a summary of what was learned using a PAR approach in research, the applicability of Bandura's self-regulation theory in audit and feedback, the value of an EDW, the weaknesses of this study, and next steps for audit and feedback research are also presented. Included in this chapter are the highlights of the background and design phase.

Literature Review

The extensive literature review for the study (though not included here) describes the current state of knowledge about audit and feedback. It also includes two separate analyses of the literature to further break down its components. Specifically, the review examines the motives for making clinical changes in inpatient settings and discusses audit and feedback in terms of definitions, data collection, purpose, and EDW. It also introduces Bandura's (1991) theoretical model for self-regulation and its application to audit and feedback. It then uses a qualitative data analysis of 36 selected articles to examine the state of the science in the literature and pertinent conclusions. It further reviews PAR and the involvement of frontline clinicians, the importance of theory, and the process of teaming and learning (Edmondson & Schein, 2012). This is followed by a further analysis of 27 articles to assess the use of theory in audit and feedback interventions. Finally, a third analysis consisting of a secondary mini-analysis of the literature based on Bandura's (1991) theory of self-regulation is performed to show how concepts from Bandura's self-regulation model can be used to assess the effectiveness of the audit and feedback literature.

PARTICIPATORY ACTION RESEARCH

PAR: Involving Clinicians in Feedback

The methodology chosen for this research is PAR. One key reason for this choice was because it integrates the frontline nurses as part of the research. More detail about PAR is given in the methods section of the chapter. In what follows, additional evidence is given to support the need to include frontline clinicians to improve patients' pain management.

Parkerton and colleagues (2009) evaluated the lessons learned from implementing TCAB in 13 hospitals from 2004 to 2008. The report began by stating: "Engagement of front-line staff is a critical component when implementing or sustaining quality improvement efforts" (Parkerton et al., 2009). The authors then emphasized that the success of changes made in quality improvement increased when supported by staff (Greenhalgh, Robert, Macfarlane, Bate, & Kyriakidou, 2004; Parker, de Pillis, Altschuler, Rubenstein, & Meredith, 2007).

Drach-Zahavy and Pud (2010) found that medication errors decreased in nursing wards when frontline nurses who administered the medication were primarily involved in analyzing and creating an action plan to reduce errors. One interesting assumption in this study was that those who analyzed and created the action plan learned the most about the medication error. Thus, it is the quality assurance or charge nurse investigating a medication error who

learns from the analysis and action plan rather than the nurses who actually administer the medications. Drach-Zahavy and Pud also reiterated that
when frontline nurses are involved in planning and implementing changes in
administering medication, these changes meet less resistance and are better
supported than if they are dictated by management (Edmondson, 2002).

The Importance of Theory

To understand the current state of knowledge on audit and feedback generally, I next selected 27 resources to help review the literature including
original research, meta-analyses, commentaries, and editorials that I felt
identified the gaps in audit and feedback research. These 27 resources initially reviewed a total of 8,220 articles for their analyses (many of the same
articles were reviewed multiple times by different researchers). Yet despite
all this research aimed at advancing and understanding audit and feedback,
a general conclusion was that little progress had been made in furthering
understanding of the process and its effectiveness (Foy et al., 2005; Ivers
et al., 2012; Jamtvedt et al., 2006; Kluger & DeNisi, 1996). This phenomenon
(a large quantity of research with little progress in understanding) may be
explained by Michie and Abraham's (2004) description of research as being
evidence inspired rather than evidence based.

What is the difference between evidence-inspired and evidence-based
research? The first has several characteristics: The intervention is vague in its
description and not reproducible, its design is not theoretically based, and a
meta-analysis of similar studies shows heterogeneity of effect sizes (Michie &
Abraham, 2004). Michie and Abraham (2004) explained these characteristics
of evidence-inspired research in evaluating a meta-analysis of studies assessing interventions to persuade pregnant women to stop smoking (Kelley,
Bond, & Abraham, 2001). The critique identified problems common to other
studies as well. One conclusion of the meta-analysis was that personal counseling may reduce the effectiveness of the smoking cessation interventions.
This is an example of a vague outcome. Is there one standard definition of
personal counseling across all studies? Were all personal counseling sessions
of the same frequency and duration? And was the content of the counseling sessions all the same? These and other questions remained unanswered.
Moreover, although most of the smoking cessation studies had significant
outcomes, the range in effect sizes was not homogeneous. Michie and
Abraham (2004) further explained that this was the result of the wide variety
of designs and procedures used in each study, failure to base design interventions on a theory, or use of a mix of theories in designing the interventions.

Similar findings were found from other research on audit and feedback. Baker and colleagues (2010), while not labeling their conclusions as evidence inspired, essentially described the same characteristics as Michie and Abraham (2004); that is, wide variation in effectiveness between studies and between the targeted behaviors within single studies, partially explained by the variety of barriers, clinical settings, and targeted behaviors, as well as lack of consistency in methods (2010, p. 12).

Clarke (1987) provided another way to view evidence-inspired versus evidence-based research by comparing research with how jig-saw puzzles are created:

> The so-called "pieces of the jig-saw" accumulate in journals [evidence inspired], despite the fact that a real jig-saw puzzle [evidence based] can only be made by taking a picture and cutting it up into pieces, not by making pieces and hoping they will form a picture. (1987, p. 35)

Research based on theory advances both the theory and the topic under study. The theory provides the "real jig-saw puzzle" view of the picture or basis for evidence. Evidence-inspired research, on the other hand, is missing the foundation that theory provides.

Kluger and DeNisi (1996) analyzed feedback interventions from 1905 to 1995 and concluded that "this research must focus on the processes induced by FIs [feedback interventions] and not on the general question of whether FIs improve performance—look at how little progress 90 years of attempts to answer the latter question have yielded" (1996, p. 278). It thus appears that the lack of theory in audit and feedback research is not a new discovery, and that those in health care research agree with this conclusion. Michie and Abraham (2004) supported the necessity of selecting an evidence-based theory: "When behaviour change interventions consist of techniques based on empirically-supported theory, then that theory provides an explanation of how the intervention works" (p. 30). Grimshaw and colleagues (2004) concurred: "Few studies provided any explicit rationale or theoretical base for the choice of intervention" (Grimshaw et al., 2004, p. 65). And Grol and colleagues (2007) spoke about the need to integrate theory into the design of intervention, commenting that:

> future studies on change interventions need to focus more on applying specific theories of change to health care. . . . the results of such research should gradually provide a better understanding of the black box of change in health care. (pp. 125–126)

Additionally, Grol and colleagues (2007) identified a lack in the study of comparative effectiveness of evidence-based theories available in health care:

> The empirical evidence of the effectiveness and feasibility of most theoretical approaches to produce the intended change in health care is limited, so it is not easy to draw conclusions about the relative superiority of any theory based on the available evidence from health care contexts. (Grol et al., 2007, p. 124)

In summarizing the research literature on audit and feedback (Foy et al., 2005), Michie, Francis, and Eccles (2008) wrote: "Without a theoretical basis, even a large literature on behaviour change interventions may offer no guidance on how to design an intervention for a new situation" (2008, p. 62). Michie, Webb, and Sniehotta (2010) later described continuing struggles in applying theory: "Theory is too often used as a 'loose framework,' to which passing reference is made, rather than as an integral part of a rigorous scientific process" (p. 1). Attempts to improve health care quality continue to suffer from lack of evidence-based theories on which to base interventions, lack of comparative effectiveness data to determine which theory might be most applicable, and lack of actual application of theory in the final design of interventions.

So what do we know after 107 years of research? We know that we need to stop researching the natural phenomenon of audit and feedback as a general or global process and to start researching the underlying components of the process. Foy and colleagues (2005) proposed a moratorium on audit and feedback interventions until we understand how and when they work. The authors suggested that the problem of too general or nonspecific audit and feedback research will be solved through "conceptualizing audit and feedback within a theoretical framework" as a way forward (p. 1). To advance from the evidence-inspired black box of outcomes to evidence-based research that will increase knowledge of the underlying processes of audit and feedback, we must interlace theory more fully into the design of the interventions in future research studies, as will be detailed in the methods section of the paper.

Understanding the importance of using theory in research is not new, but how to apply theory in designing interventions to change behavior within research may be misunderstood. Michie and Prestwich (2010) proposed a model of how to ensure that theory is an integral part of designing interventions in one's research, beginning with choosing an appropriate theory. According to Michie and colleagues, it is important to select a theory that is based on how to change behavior rather than explain behavior (2008). For instance, Ajzen's

Table 4.1 *Theory-Coding Schema to Guide Evidence-Based Intervention Designs*

Category	Description
1	Is the theory mentioned?
2	Are the relevant theoretical constructs targeted?
3	Is the theory used to select recipients or tailor interventions?
4	Are the relevant theoretical constructs measured?
5	Is the theory tested?
6	Is the theory refined?

(1991) theory of planned behavior and Bandura's (1997) social cognitive theory are used in behavioral research, but Bandura's theory is about designing interventions to change behaviors, whereas Ajzen's theory is used to understand behavior to change it, but doesn't describe how to design interventions to change the behavior. This is one reason why Bandura's (1991) social cognitive theory of self-regulation was chosen to guide this research.

The next step involves integrating the chosen theory into the intervention design. Michie and Prestwich (2010) validated a tool that can be used to ensure that an intervention is theory based. This tool can be used in multiple ways either in designing theory-based interventions or evaluating completed research if it is theory based. For my research, the theory-coding schema, which is described in further detail in the methods section of the paper, is used to help design theory–based interventions. The theory-coding schema is made up of 19 items organized into six categories, as seen in Table 4.1.

Michie and Prestwich (2010) also provided further detail on each category and related items. The interventions for the present study will follow this theory-coding schema to ensure that theory has been integrated into each step of the intervention design.

In sum, an overview of evidence-inspired and evidence-based research has been given to explain why cumulative progress is lagging in the audit and feedback area. A review of existing research conclusions on audit and feedback, and more broadly on changing health care behaviors, has revealed a common theme of the importance of integrating theory into the development of interventions.

Teaming and Learning

In 2009, a local hospital system implemented a protocol for nurses to establish pain goals with patients. But despite the approval of the protocol, compliance was extremely low. To try to improve compliance, a feedback report was made available to hospitals, the report could be run at any time via the intranet, and data could be viewed at the hospital, nurse unit, or nurse level. Within 8 months, the system averaged 70% to 75% compliance on establishing pain goals. Joint Commission auditors were impressed by the improvement and feedback reports. Yet the only thing that improved during this time was the performance on documenting pain goals. Patients' perceptions of how well their pain was managed during their hospital stay remained the same over the 8 months and did not improve. What this project demonstrated was that it takes more than feedback, even if optimally delivered, to improve patient care. In this case, the purpose of creating feedback was to improve nursing documentation to meet The Joint Commission's requirements for addressing pain. Yet the question remained: How could the feedback be used to improve patient outcomes?

One answer may be found in the research of Dr. Amy C. Edmondson, a Harvard Novartis Leadership and Management professor. Over the past 20 years, her research has crossed many disciplines, from analyzing medical errors in hospitals to examining the failed space shuttle Columbia mission. Specifically, her research has focused on leadership's influence on learning and collaboration and innovation in teams and organizations (Harvard Business School, 2012). Edmondson and Schein's (2012) book *Teaming: How Organizations Learn, Innovate, and Compete in the Knowledge Industry* describes a framework for how the environment can integrate with audit and feedback to improve patient outcomes.

Edmondson and Schein (2012) found that collecting data and including the participation of frontline clinicians improved patient outcomes. As Edmondson stated, "My research has found that a lack of access to data on failures is the most important barrier to managers learning from them" (2012, p. 173). But if an EDW were utilized, access to data would not be as big a barrier to managers or to frontline providers.

Edmondson and Schein (2012) emphasized the key differences between execution-as-efficiency and execution-as-learning and established the importance of including employees in the process. The three most important differences between the two approaches are in the roles of leadership, feedback, and employees. In execution-as-efficiency, leaders supply the answer, feedback is one-way in the direction of the employees, and employee input is discouraged. In execution-as-learning, leaders create an environment for learning, feedback is two-way, and employee engagement is critical. Thus, these are two highly contrasting styles of leadership. Edmonson and Schein believed that execution-as-efficiency was the predominant form of management but improving patient care required a transition to execution-as-learning.

Not all hospital failures require the same approach to be solved. But it is important to understand the different types of failure first before describing the approaches. Edmondson and Schein (2012) categorized three types of failures: preventable, complex, and intelligent. Preventable failures occur in well-defined processes and happen because of a lack of skill or behavior or because of insufficient support. An example of a preventable failure would be failing to raise the bed rails on fall-risk patients when putting them back to bed. Preventable failures often result from deviating from the standard of care (Edmondson & Schein, 2012).

Complex failures are related to novel interactions that typically produce uncertainty in the work setting (Edmondson & Schein, 2012). Currently many hospitals are struggling to meet the government's requirement to improve scores on the HCAHPS survey. The HCAHPS assesses various patient perceptions for care received during a hospital stay. Specifically, it has been difficult to improve patients' perception of how their pain was managed. Unlike improving nurses' compliance with a clinical practice guideline, this measure requires changing patients' perceptions on how well their pain was managed, and despite multiple interventions, there does not appear to be a silver bullet for solving this problem. Thus, improving HCAHPS qualifies as a complex failure.

The last type of failure is intelligent failure. Intelligent failures are judged as good because what is learned from them helps in finding the solution (Edmondson & Schein, 2012). Pharmaceutical companies, inventors, and medical research (such as oncology) fit this category. Learning from failure is the goal in these situations.

Edmondson and Schein (2012) proposed three different approaches to analyze and resolve each of the three types of failures. Preventable failures are associated with procedures that are well defined and where the goal is to duplicate them with little variation. Because these are typically high-volume procedures, total quality management (TQM) and statistical analysis are well suited to detect variation. In this case, audit and feedback would focus on highlighting the failures detected by TQM and statistical analysis.

In situations where the failure is complex and novel, TQM and statistical analysis are not good approaches; instead, the best method is to pull together specialized individuals with diverse experience (Edmondson & Schein, 2012). Using the HCAHPS example mentioned earlier, the best solution would be to pull together a diverse group of specialized individuals, such as nurses, nurse's aides, clerks, social workers, physicians, behavioral psychologists, pain specialists, patients, and management, to discuss and analyze how best to improve patients' perceptions of pain. Critical to bringing this group together is the inclusion of data abstraction and an analysis specialist, who could facilitate fact finding and give feedback to the group. It is also important that a leader or facilitator be used to ensure that the group works together and to handle differing opinions.

When conditions involve intelligent failures and call for innovation, the approach is similar to that for complex failures, but here, the need focuses on a detailed, systematic analysis with highly skilled individuals (Edmondson & Schein, 2012). In this approach, the team wants to learn from a failure as quickly as possible without overlooking any potential cause for it. Edmondson and Schein (2012) provide the example of an experimental drug that failed a series of trials; instead of assuming that the failure was related to the drug, the physician did a thorough investigation and discovered that in fact it was related to patients who had low folic acid levels. Administering folic acid supplements to the patient mitigated the failure.

In conclusion, Edmondson and Schein (2012) have shown that different approaches are required to resolve different types of failure. They have also validated the need for audit and feedback of data and for creating work teams of frontline employees. Although their book is full of insightful research on concepts of leadership and teaming that are important to this study, here I have described only that information that is critical to the design of this study and that has added to the latest evidence base on audit and feedback and improvement of patient outcomes.

Secondary Analysis Based on Bandura's (1991) Self-Regulation Theory

As noted earlier, one of the primary meta-analyses on audit and feedback was a 2006 Cochrane Review, which came from the Effective Practice and Organization of Care review group of the Cochrane Collaboration. In this review, Jamtvedt and colleagues analyzed 118 studies using the following criteria: intensity of the audit and feedback, complexity of the targeted behavior, seriousness of the outcome, and level of baseline compliance and study quality. The authors concluded that audit and feedback could be effective in improving clinicians' practice and that the effects were typically small to medium. Yet in summary, the authors also concluded that "it is striking how little can be discerned about the effects of audit and feedback based on the 118 trials included in this review" (2006, p. 22). The authors then made four recommendations on how future trials could determine the effectiveness of audit and feedback, which are as follows:

1. Trials should be well designed, conducted, and reported.
2. Because outcomes have only small-to-medium effects, the trials should be adequately powered.

3. Process evaluations should be well designed to provide insights into the varying degrees of effectiveness of the audit and feedback procedures.
4. Head-to-head comparisons should be made of different ways of performing audit and feedback.

These recommendations could be considered general guidelines for doing quality research. Yet more could be learned from these studies that cannot be concluded from a quantitative meta-analysis alone if they were analyzed with the guidance of a theory. I therefore undertook a mini-analysis of these studies by measuring concepts identified in Bandura's (1991) system of self-regulation and Edmondson and Schein's (2012) concept of teaming. Of all 118 research studies used in the 2006 Cochrane Review, only 24 had received a rank of high quality (Jamtvedt et al., 2006). For the mini-analysis I loaded PDF files of all 24 high-quality studies into ATLAS.ti and then used an inductive approach over the next 6 months to analyze the data. I coded and recoded each study multiple times, in the process identifying concepts from Bandura's system of self-regulation. Table 4.2 displays the final list of concepts, which will be described in detail.

Each study was assessed on whether the design of the intervention was based on a theory. Including a theory in the design gave credence to the chosen approach of the intervention, thus showing how important theory is in designing such studies.

For each study, the number of different interventions it used was counted. Types of intervention included audit and feedback, education sessions, and study support. Study support was defined as the study team hiring someone to work with a site or recruiting a local opinion leader from the site to assist in the study. The types of intervention could also be aligned with teaming, valuation, and referential performance.

Table 4.2 *Concepts Used to Code Studies*

Concept	Definition
Theory	Whether the study's intervention was based on a theory
Intervention	Type of intervention(s) used in the study
Approach	Passive: Unsolicited feedback given to recipient to review Active: Individuals identified who were responsible for engaging intended recipients in reviewing feedback
Frequency	How many times study participants interacted with interventions
Duration	How long the intervention lasted
Level	Level of feedback specificity, whether by individual or group

The approach of the intervention defined the relationship between the interventions and the study participants. In passive approaches, the interventions were acting on the study participants, whereas active approaches allowed interventions to act on the participants and the participants to act on the interventions. This concept is tightly aligned with teaming.

Frequency of the interventions was defined as the number of times the recipients had some type of interaction with any intervention. If they attended an educational session, received two phone call consults, received feedback twice, and had reminders in their patients' charts, the total frequency would be at least six. Frequency was aligned with teaming, regularity, and proximity.

Duration of the intervention was defined as the time from the beginning to the end of the study. This was measured in calendar months or years. Duration could influence teaming, valuation, regularity, proximity, and performance attribution.

Level of feedback specified whether the feedback was given at the individual level or at a higher level such as a site. Site level was defined as either a group of physicians practicing together or all physicians in a hospital. Level of feedback was aligned with teaming, informativeness, performance attribution, referential performance, and valuation.

Table 4.3 displays the analysis of the 24 reviewed studies (see Appendix 4A for a more detailed explanation). An overall outcome for each study was given based on the magnitude of each study's effect. Specifically, outcomes showing no significant differences between groups were labeled ND, those showing significant differences in some variables but not all were labeled D, and those reporting significant differences between groups for the primary outcome were labeled SD. All 24 studies were quantitative and measured success by showing significant differences between the control and intervention groups.

Of the 24 studies, 21 made no mention of theory in the design of the study or intervention. The three studies that did mention a theory did so only in passing, giving little detail about the theory or how it was used to design the study or intervention. Thus, theory did not form a significant part of any of the 24 high-quality studies.

Of these 24 studies, 15 used onsite support as one of the interventions. Onsite support was identified as support by staff, physicians, registered nurses, or clinicians, and as either external or provided by a local opinion leader. External support meant that someone from the research team or hired by the team was at the study site helping with the interventions. A local opinion leader supported the interventions at the site in the same way except that he or she originated from the site. Of interest is that seven of the eight studies that used a local opinion leader had significant results.

Table 4.3 *Analysis of Audit and Feedback Research*

Author	Intervention(s)	Approach	Frequency	Duration	Level	Outcome
Baker	Audits	Passive	1	1 year	Site	ND
Ferguson	MD(L)/audits/education	Active	3	18 months	Site	SD
Goff	Audits	Passive	3	3 years	Site	ND
Hayes	MD(L) and/or audits	Active	1	4 months	Site	ND
Hendryx	Clinicians(E)/audit	Active	4	1 year	Site	D
Hillman	Audits	Passive	3	18 months	Site	ND
Katz	Staff(E)/audit	Active	5	1 year	Provider	D
Kerse	Education/audit	Active	3	1 year	Provider	D
Kinsinger	MD(E)/audit	Active	2 +	18 months	Provider	D
Lemelin	RN(E)/education/audit	Active	2 +	18 months	Practice	SD
Leviton	MD(L)/education/audit	Active	3	1 year	Site	SD
Lomas	MD(L)/education/audit	Active	?	2 years	?	SD
Manfredi	Staff(E)/education/audit	Active	4	2 years	Provider	SD
O'Connell	Audit	Passive	4	2 years	Provider	ND
Primlott	Audit/education	Passive	3	6 months	Provider	ND
Quinley	Audits/Staff(E)	Active	3	1 year	Provider	D
Sauaia	MD(E)/educ. & or audit	Active	1	6 months	Provider	ND
Sondergaard	Audit	Passive	2	6 months	Site	ND
Sondergaard	Audit	Passive	2	6 months	Site	ND
Soumerai	MD(L)/education/audit	Active	2 +	10 months	Site	SD
Thompson	Staff(L)/education/audit	Active	13	1 year	Site	SD
Verstappen	Staff(E)/education/audit	Active	3	6 months.	Provider	D
Vingerhoets	Audit	Passive	1	15 months.	Provider	ND
Wells	Staff(L)/education/audit	Active	12	1 year	Provider	SD

ND, no difference; D, difference; SD, significant difference; MD, physician; RN, registered nurse; E, external support; L, local opinion leader.

Nine of 24 studies were coded as using a passive approach to feedback. The main intervention used in these studies was mailing letters or posting audit results in the offices of the intended unsolicited recipients. Feedback using the passive approach did not produce any difference or significant difference between the control and intervention groups, even when some participants were paid by the study for improved performance (Hillman & Ripley, 1999). The advantages of passive feedback are its simplicity and lower intervention costs, but despite these benefits, it appears that if feedback is unsolicited, it will go unnoticed.

In contrast, 13 of the 15 studies using an active approach showed a difference or significant difference in their outcomes. The two studies that did not see positive results appeared to have design flaws in their intervention. In the study by Hayes and colleagues (2001), the time between intervention and remeasurement was only 4 months, which did not allow sufficient time to disseminate the feedback to all hospital physicians or for it to take effect. In the other study, Sauaia and colleagues (2000) provided feedback about standard of care for ischemic heart disease through an in-hospital education presentation. Although the presentation sought to change physician practice in prescribing medications for ischemic heart patients, few physicians attended. Thus, although the interventions in these two studies appeared to provide good education and feedback, the logistics of disseminating the feedback effectively to physicians was a barrier to both studies.

Frequency of interventions also revealed no differences in the passive approach, but this probably had more to do with the passivity of the approach than with the frequency. On the other hand, an increase in frequency in the active approach showed a trend toward significant differences. The frequency range in the difference (D) group was 3 to 5, and in the significant difference (SD) group 3 to 15. Thus, it appears intuitive to say that the more intense (the higher the frequency of feedback) an intervention is, the more effective it will be.

Examining the range and median of the duration for each of the three groups (ND, D, and SD) showed a trend whereby the longer the duration, the more effective the intervention. The interventions of the ND group ranged from 6 to 36 months with a median of 9; those of the D group ranged from 6 to 12 months with a median of 12; and those of the SD group ranged from 10 to 24 months with a median of 15. Although showing the range and median of the passive groups (ND) is interesting, increasing the duration did not appear to improve outcomes. But in the active groups, the longer the duration, the better the outcomes. A good example is the study by Hayes and colleagues (2001), which used an active approach, had a short 4-month duration, and produced a result showing no difference between the control and intervention groups.

Looking at the level of feedback among the three outcomes groups revealed a mixed result. In the ND group, audit and feedback was provided four times at the provider level and six times at the practice level. The SD group gave feedback at the provider level twice and practice level four times. The D group showed the only trend toward a possible difference, with feedback given at the provider level five times and once at the practice level. With such mixed results among all the groups, it is challenging to make any observations.

This secondary analysis on the 24 high-quality studies from the 2006 Cochrane Review (Jamtvedt et al., 2006) was performed to demonstrate the plausibility of using concepts from Bandura's (1991) social cognitive theory of self-regulation and Edmonson and Schein's (2012) teaming approach in assessing the effectiveness of interventions in influencing clinician behavior so as to improve patient outcomes. Moreover, as this analysis was nearing completion, an update on the original 2006 Cochrane Review published in June 2012 (Ivers et al., 2012) further supported its conclusion. According to the review:

> feedback may be more effective when baseline performance is low, when the source is a supervisor or senior colleague, when it is provided more than once, when it is provided both verbally and written, and when it includes both measurable targets and an action plan. (p. 33)

Feedback coming from a supervisor or senior colleague supports the use of an active approach. Feedback provided more than once and in multiple ways supports the use of multiple interventions, with the goal of increasing the number of times that recipients interact with those interventions. Feedback that includes both measurable targets and an action plan is another way of making it informative. Yet to understand better how clinician behavior can be influenced to improve patient outcomes requires research using a theory-based approach in designing the intervention, such as Bandura's (1991) system of self-regulation or Edmondson and Schein's (2012) process of teaming.

One final conclusion found in Ivers and colleagues' (2012) Cochrane Review is the issue of the cost and time required to create effective audit and feedback interventions. The authors stated that "pragmatic consideration needs to be given to additional costs associated with providing feedback more frequently, providing both verbal and written feedback, and using a supervisor or colleague to provide feedback, since these features may entail additional costs" (2012, p. 33). The cost of interventions such as audit and feedback, educational seminars, and recruitment and use of local opinion leaders remains a barrier. Yet such barriers related to performing audit and feedback and doing so frequently would be largely mitigated by using an EDW to abstract data from EMRs and making it available to anyone given access to the feedback report. The cost to hire and train a nurse to do manual data abstraction for well-known programs like NSQIP is about $90,000 a year, but how much that nurse can manually abstract on a daily basis is limited. This, in turn, limits the scalability of the manual program in looking at additional populations of patients, the timeliness of results, and their availability in disseminating feedback to recipients. Although there are upfront costs in starting an EDW and automating the audit and feedback process, scalability is not an issue, feedback reports are updated at least daily if not more often, and the feedback is available to anyone with access to the report on the intranet. In the end, the costs of performing audit and feedback manually or by automation are about the same, but the potential upsides to using an EDW warrants this research.

CONCLUSION

Because of the government's shift to value-based purchasing, hospitals and providers face a new challenge in how to deliver planned care that avoids incidental events and improves the value of care perceived by patients. Audit and feedback has a long history as an intervention used in health care to improve outcomes but comes with mixed results. A key finding of the analysis of audit and feedback is the lack of theory used in designing interventions. This literature review shows that Albert Bandura's social cognitive theory of self-regulation is a good theory to follow in designing interventions of audit and feedback.

Another important finding is that of including nurses in interventions to improve patient outcomes. Frontline nurses not only need to be active in this process but also need an integrated approach to effectively improve patients' pain management care during their hospital stay.

The EDW is a technology that can improve audit and feedback, designed following Bandura's social cognitive theory of self-regulation and supportive of an integrated approach to improving patients' pain management care. This research will evaluate how well the EDW achieves these objectives.

METHODOLOGY

The overarching purpose of this study is to compare two audit and feedback processes that report on nurses' documentation compliance with pain management protocols. Although it is concerned with pain management, the study also presents a novel audit and feedback process that could be applied to any hospital protocol where documentation compliance is measured.

This chapter describes the current peer-reviewed audit process and compares it with the process I have developed for this study to provide nurses with feedback on pain documentation performance. It then explains the three pain assessments that will be audited for this study using the new process, followed by the study's aims and research questions, method, data analysis, limitations, and anticipated challenges.

The MDR and EDW Audit Processes

The following paragraphs compare the manual audit process known as the medical document review (MDR), which is currently in use, with the EDW audit process that was developed for this study. This includes an analysis comparing the audit outcomes of both processes in charting pain management goals (PMGs) and pain intensity scores (PISs) for the last 8 months of 2012.

The MDR Process

The MDR was created at this hospital for four purposes. The first was to educate staff about regulatory, accreditation, and hospital requirements for medical record documentation. Second, the MDR was to provide a single method by which all audits can be performed within the hospital. Third, the MDR was expected to furnish documentation for regulatory and accreditation agencies when required. Finally, the MDR was to provide a way to collect data to support hospital goals and improve performance. The MDR program includes a list of questions used to audit nursing documentation compliance with the hospital's clinical practice guidelines. Clinicians manually look at the EMR of a given patient to judge whether the documentation was done correctly and then enter their findings into the MDR program. Data from the MDR audit are then summarized, and a report is made available on the intranet to show the nursing units' documentation compliance with the hospital's clinical practice guidelines.

All nurses on the medical–surgical unit currently perform one manual audit, consisting of 19 questions, each month either on one of their own patient's medical records or on those of another nurse's patient. The nurse logs into the MDR application, enters the patient's encounter number, and then manually reviews the EMR to answer the manual audit questions.

Comparison of the MDR and EDW Processes

Figure 4.1 illustrates the basic flow of the MDR and the prototype EDW processes. Although both processes look similar in their flow, there is a significant difference in how the audit portion is completed. As noted above, the MDR audit is performed manually on a sample representation of the population by the nurses on the unit. The prototype EDW audit process used in this study replaces the manual audit with automated data queries that pull data from the EMR each night and summarize them in the EDW. The following day, the updated audit and feedback reports are uploaded on the intranet and made available for frontline nurses to review. The difference between the two processes resides primarily in the manner in which the audit is done and in the richness of the data pulled by the EDW queries.

Another illustration of the differences between the manual and automated methods for abstracting data on pain documentation can be seen in an analysis of audit results at the hospital under study for the last 8 months of 2012. The analysis compared the audit results using the MDR method with those using the prototype EDW method in examining compliance with documenting a PMG and a PIS within 12 hours of a patient's admission. Table 4.4 displays the results of the analysis.

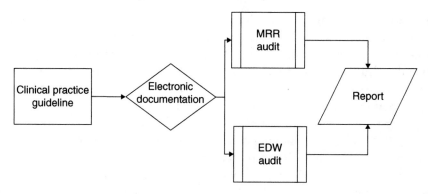

Figure 4.1 *MDR and EDW audit processes.*

Table 4.4 *2012 Audit Results of Pain Documentation Using Manual and Automated Methods*

Audit of pain documentation	May	Jun	Jul	Aug	Sep	Oct	Nov	Dec
Total MDR PMG audits	7	52	20	40	64	22	39	19
Total PMG documented	7	46	19	38	54	16	33	19
MDR audit PMG	100%	88%	95%	95%	84%	73%	85%	100%
Total EDW PMG audits	210	207	191	203	187	215	189	248
Total PMG documented	181	173	169	182	145	182	167	208
EDW audit PMG	86%	84%	88%	90%	78%	85%	88%	84%
Total MDR PIS audits	4	27	10	19	32	11	20	9
Total PIS documented	3	26	10	16	30	10	20	9
MDR audit PIS	75%	96%	100%	84%	94%	91%	100%	100%
Total EDW PIS audits	232	207	191	203	177	215	189	243
Total PIS documented	222	202	189	200	176	213	185	241
EDW audit PIS	96%	98%	99%	99%	99%	99%	98%	99%

MDR, medical document review; PMG, pain management goal; EDW, enterprise data warehouse; PIS, pain intensity score.

What Table 4.4 does not show is the small sample on which MDR is based. The MDR sample for documenting PMG as a proportion of the total population of patients or the MDR audit rate for PMG ranged from a low of 3% in May 2012 (7 out of 210 total) to a high of 34% in September 2012 (64 out of 187 total). The MDR sample for documenting PIS as a proportion of the total population of patients or the MDR audit rate for PIS ranged from a low of 2% in May (4 out of 232 total) to a high of 18% in September (32 out of 177 total). But sampling rates such as these are too low, producing high variations that negatively affect the reliability of the results, which may be interpreted incorrectly. It would be difficult to determine from looking at the overall monthly trends of nurse manual audits for PMG and PIS documentation whether any monthly rate was within normal variation or was truly a signal that the process was out of control as a result of bad sampling. In contrast, the EDW audit looks at 100% of all PMG and PIS documentation and is nearly 100% reliable in showing whether compliance with documenting the PMG and PIS from month to month is within normal variation.

Both the PMG and PIS documentation requirements are defined by hospital protocols. The fact that the EDW audit is nearly 100% reliable and does not use subjective but rather objective reasoning to determine whether the pain documentation is in compliance with the pain protocols strengthens its validity.

Pain Assessments Used in This Study

In addition to auditing the initial PMG and PIS, this study will include two additional assessments. Preintervention–postintervention opioid assessments, which have not been measured so far, will provide a good baseline for the newly introduced audit and feedback measurements. Table 4.5 provides a description of each assessment.

Blood pressure (BP), heart rate (HR), and respiratory rate (RR) are objective measures of how well patients are maintaining these natural functions on their own. The no sedative effects, anxiolysis, moderate sedation, or unconsciousness (NAMDU) scale, which is a subjective measurement of a patient's sedation level made by a nurse, ranges from no sedative effect to unconsciousness. The PMG is a number ranging from 1 to 10 that the nurse and patient/family establish; the object is to select a number that allows the patient to be comfortable and functioning although the patient may still have some pain. The PIS is a subjective measure reported by the patient of the level of pain the patient is currently experiencing; although this score uses various scales, the results all register between 1 and 10.

The admission PMG and PIS documentation normally has a higher rate of compliance because there is a 12-hour window for these to be documented. But because the PMG documentation is not as routine as the PIS, it will be missed more often, and the nurse may forget to document a new PMG if there is a change in patient status; for instance, a patient just returned from surgery requires documentation of a new PMG.

Table 4.5 *Required Pain Assessments, Frequency of Assessment, and Measured Metrics*

Assessment	Frequency	Measured Metrics
Arrival PMG and PIS	Within 12 hours of admission	PMG, PIS
Opioid preintervention	Within 12 hours before initiating therapy	BP, HR, RR, NAMDU, PIS
Opioid postintervention	1 hour after administration	RR, NAMDU, PIS

PMG, pain management goal; PIS, pain intensity score; BP, blood pressure; HR, heart rate; RR, respiratory rate; NAMDU, no sedative effects, anxiolysis, moderate sedation, unconsciousness.

The preassessment documentation checks whether the BP, HR, RR, PIS, and NAMDU are charted within 12 hours of giving an opioid. Compliance with documenting the preassessment is expected to be high because nurses have up to 12 hours after administering the opioid to complete documentation. The compliance rate regarding postassessment RR and NAMDU, however, is likely to be lower because these are to be reassessed within an hour of opioid administration. The postassessment is easy to overlook when a single nurse may be giving multiple opioids to multiple patients during his or her shift.

Table 4.6 lists the 2012 performance for documenting these three pain assessments in the medical–surgical unit under study.

Overall, the preintervention and pain intensity goal and score documentation compliance were above 90%, whereas the postopioid assessment was very low in the range of 31% to 33%. The pain documentation average is calculated by averaging the three documented assessments (arrival, preassessment, and postassessment), and provides an overall performance measure of how well the unit documents pain assessments. When measuring overall performance in pain documentation in the three areas, overall the nursing unit is compliant in charting 63% of the time. The purpose of having clinical practice guidelines that dictate clinical documentation (like pain assessments) is to ensure the patient is receiving optimal care. In this case, it is an assumption that pain documentation compliance represents

Table 4.6 *2012 Compliance With Pain Documentation Standard Expectations*

Documentation	Documented/Total Expected	%
Arrival PMG	2,114/2,457	86
Arrival PIS	2,409/2,457	98
Preassessment HR	30,753/32,386	95
Preassessment BP	30,755/32,386	95
Preassessment RR	30,980/32,386	96
Preassessment NAMDU	26,308/32,386	81
Preassessment PIS	30,960/32,386	96
Postassessment RR	10,723/32,386	33
Postassessment NAMDU	10,162/32,386	31
Pain documentation average	42,654/67,229	63

PMG, pain management goal; PIS, pain intensity score; HR, heart rate; BP, blood pressure; RR, respiratory rate; NAMDU, no sedative effects, anxiolysis, moderate sedation, unconsciousness.

optimal care, which currently stands at 63%. In other words the patients on this medical–surgical unit get optimal pain management care of 63% during their stay in the hospital.

Study Aims and Research Questions: Baseline

In any comparison study, a baseline must be established. The first aim of this study is to understand nurses' perceptions of the purpose, benefits, and drawbacks of the current MDR audit and feedback process. This involves establishing their general overall knowledge of the two audit and feedback processes (MDR and EDW prototype). The nurses will be asked research questions 1 and 2 at the beginning of the study for the MDR process and, again, at the end of the study for the EDW prototype process.

1. Research question 1: According to the nurses, what is the purpose of the audit and feedback process?
2. Research question 2: What do nurses perceive to be the benefits and drawbacks of the audit and feedback process?

The second aim of this study is to develop and describe a prototype process, based on Bandura's (1991) social cognitive theory of self-regulation, for using the EDW to create an automated audit and feedback report for pain management protocols in a collaborative and participatory setting with frontline nurses and then analyze what was learned throughout the process. Research questions 3 and 4 address these issues:

3. Research question 3: What was collaboratively learned in creating audit and feedback with frontline nurses that would improve the future development of this prototype?
4. Research question 4: What changes (format, content, delivery) need to be made from the initial to final version of the feedback, and why?

The final aim focuses on comparing and contrasting the peer-reviewed MDR and the collaborative automated EDW process for creating audit and feedback with respect to documentation outcomes and nurses' preferences, if any. Research questions 5 and 6 deal with these issues:

5. Research question 5: Does charting compliance with pain assessments (Table 4.6) improve using the sequential versions of the audit and feedback prototype process?

6. Research question 6: What do nurses think about the relative merits, if any, in using the prototype audit and feedback process over the peer-reviewed MDR process?

DESIGN

In the 24 studies reviewed by Jamtvedt and colleagues (2006), most used variations of the pretest–posttest design O_1 X O_2. This study's design is similar to methods used within the health care setting for making continuous improvements in quality. Typically, when a problem has been identified in health care, a small group of key individuals will perform multiple cycles of "plan, do, study, act" (PDSA) until a satisfactory outcome is met. The design notation looks like this: O_1 X_1 O_2 X_2 O_3 X_3 O_4 . . . , where each X_x represents a modification to the audit and feedback per input from the clinicians. This is an ongoing repetitive process, and through time, fewer and fewer changes will be needed. The same design will be used for this research. An analogy that may be helpful is that of improving the design of an airplane while flying it. In this study I will be analyzing and developing the design of clinician performance feedback while at the same time seeking to improve documentation compliance.

Participatory Action Research

Trying to improve a complex issue like inpatient pain management requires a methodology that involves everyone as a researcher. One such method is PAR, which is defined somewhat differently, depending on the field in which it is used. The preferred definition for this study is taken from the field of organizational and professional development, as given by Argyris and Schon (1989):

> Action research takes its cues—its questions, puzzles, and problems—from the perceptions of practitioners within particular, local practice contexts and builds descriptions and theories within the practice context then tests them there through intervention experiments. (p. 86)

The PAR method has two important elements regarding participation that differ substantially from other methodologies. First, the primary investigator (PI) is doing research not on the participants but, rather, with them (i.e., as co-researchers). In other words, the co-researchers are an active part of the study. In this study, co-researchers will include primarily the staff nurses on the unit as well as nurse's aides and the nursing leadership. In previous PAR studies, co-researchers have helped carry out actual coding of data, decided how funds were to be used in research, and defined interventions (Herr & Anderson, 2005). In this research, the co-researchers will help in developing the feedback and will share their perspectives on its effectiveness. Everyone participating in the research will have a vested self-interest in its outcome.

The second element that differs in PAR is the role of the PI. In other methodologies, typically, PIs must be careful to remain at a safe distance and not influence the research under study. In PAR, on the other hand, the PI or other researchers have a choice to be either internal or external to the study. For this project, I (the PI) will be considered an insider, actively working with and giving input into the study. My interest in looking at feedback and its effect on patient outcomes comes from my own experience as a nurse, charge nurse, nurse manager, and nurse informaticist, so I have already served in the roles of those I will include as co-researchers. From my perspective, I believe that feedback is critical to improving the outcomes of patients, but in many ways, this element is missing in nursing today. I have often wondered what Florence Nightingale would have done without feedback in 1855 while caring for wounded soldiers at Scutari. Would she have been able to decrease preventable mortality significantly without performance feedback?

Application of Bandura's (1991) Self-Regulation Theory in Designing Feedback

This study's purpose and goals will require PAR for its success. The following describes how I have combined Bandura's (1991) theoretical framework with a PAR approach to research and create nursing performance feedback with the goal of understanding how valuable nurses find various elements in the feedback. As described earlier, the initial feedback design was based on Bandura's (1991) social cognitive theory of self-regulation. The audit and feedback will be performed on the degree to which the nurses' documentation complies with the hospital's clinical pain management protocol.

The following describes the preintervention metric of BP for each part of the model listed in Appendix 4B to show how the feedback is based on Bandura (1991). To represent informativeness, the nurse will see his or her rate of documenting BP before that of all pain interventions; the same metric is also calculated for both the nursing unit and the hospital. These metrics will be displayed as a ratio of actual documented BP to documentation opportunities. The nurse will also see his or her performance compared with unit and hospital goals. To show progress over time, the trend of the nurse's documentation of BP before an intervention over the previous 12 months will be displayed on a chart.

How much the nurse's charting contributes to the overall unit and hospital goals is shown next to those goals. The attribution ratio is determined by dividing the nurse's BP documentation opportunities by either the unit's or hospital's total opportunities.

The display for referential performance showed similar metrics for BP documented before an intervention, but now the data show the nurse's performance compared with that of his or her peers. There will be multiple ways to sort the data based on the columns.

To verify the accuracy of the data, nurses will see the details regarding documenting their BP readings. For example, if there were 30 opportunities to document BP before a pain intervention, the nurse would see the details for each one, including a patient identifier for looking up the patient in the EMR and validating the audit and feedback report.

Regularity is represented by allowing nurses to access the audit and feedback report at any time while at work. The nurses will be shown how they can access the report on the intranet and will be sent a weekly e-mail with a link to the report. So, although I cannot force the nurses to view the report with regularity, I can provide them the opportunity to do so.

Proximity will be used in two contexts. First, if a nurse documents a patient's BP before a pain intervention on one day, on the following day the audit and feedback report will show that the nurse was compliant in following the protocol. The time between documenting the BP and showing the result on the audit and feedback report is proximate. The second context of proximity is what is being measured on the audit and feedback report. Measuring the documentation of BP before a pain intervention is more proximate to the nurse than to the number of patients who are hypotensive after a pain intervention.

All nurses who look at the audit and feedback report have the option to provide feedback (valuation) on the report. The feedback can include suggestions for improvement, complaints that they do not like it, or indicators of the value of the report. The ability to accept feedback from the nurses will not only help improve the report but also provide data to show whether they judge the report to be of value overall.

In addition to giving nurses their own personal feedback, these same measures will be duplicated at a facility and system level.

Setting

The hospital under study is a 97-bed, Level 4 community hospital located in the Intermountain West. Hospital services consist of an emergency department, inpatient and outpatient surgical services, an inpatient adult medical–surgical unit, an adult intensive care unit, labor and delivery, a mother and baby care unit, a special care nursery, and an inpatient children's unit. The hospital opened in 2009 with a focus on patient-centered care and offers a blend of high-tech and high-touch medicine.

Human Subjects' Protections and Considerations

The main participants in this research will be hospital leadership and nursing staff on the medical–surgical unit. No identifying information about participants such as name, employee ID, or address will be included in the final dissertation. All interviews will be digitally recorded by audio and maintained on a digital recorder kept in a locked location until transferred to a password-protected file on a password-protected computer in a locked office. Once interviews are transferred to the computer, the actual recording will be erased from the digital recorder.

It is not required to collect or analyze identifiable personal health information from patients in this research. Patient account numbers will appear on the audit and feedback report, which is password protected and can be viewed only on the hospital's intranet by those clinicians who have access to the report.

Participants can be identified in the audit and feedback data, access to which is determined by hospital leadership. Any decision about how to use the identifiable audit and feedback information is under the direction of hospital leadership. This information has always been available to hospital leadership through manual chart audits, and the same information will now be available in a different form.

Any e-mail correspondence between the study co-researchers and me may be used for this study's analysis. All e-mail information used for analysis will be de-identified before being transcribed to a password-protected study file on my computer. All e-mails will be deleted once the information has been transcribed

Informed consent will be obtained at the hospital level as agreed upon by hospital leadership. All study co-researchers will receive a written description of the study, listing its purpose and their options for participating. At any time during the study, if a co-researcher chooses not to be included in the research, the researcher simply e-mails a request to the PI, and the researcher's information will be removed from the feedback report and the researcher will no longer be interviewed or e-mailed questions.

Every time I digitally record audio conversations with participants, I will disclose beforehand the purpose and intent in recording this information. During the transcription process, any identifiable participant information will be de-identified.

Protocol

The study will last a total of 14 weeks divided into four stages, shown in Table 4.7. The following describes how data will be collected and presents the highlights of what happens in each stage.

Qualitative data will be collected in three ways. The preferred method is to make digital recordings whenever I am talking with nurses in group meetings or in one-on-one conversations. Whenever digital recording is not optimal, I will use field notes to record conversations I have with staff. The final method of collecting qualitative data will be through an e-mail link labeled *suggestion to improve feedback* within the prototype feedback report. Table 4.8 lists the various meetings, interviews, and e-mail correspondences to be used in all phases of collecting data.

Quantitative data include documentation performance vis-à-vis required hospital pain assessments as seen in Table 4.5 and the frequency with which nurses access and view the prototype audit and feedback report. All these data will be captured electronically in the EMR and summarized either in the EDW or from metrics generated about the prototype audit and feedback report.

In Stage 1 of the study I will attend all five meetings listed in Table 4.8. After giving an overall introduction to my research to each group, I will

Table 4.7 *Study Stages*

Stage	Duration	Topic
1	2 weeks	Baseline MDR
2	4 weeks	Initial pain report feedback
3	4 weeks	First revision
4	4 weeks	Final revision

Table 4.8 *Data Collection Sources*

Audience	Purpose	Type	Frequency
Leadership	Unit leadership coordination	Meeting	Monthly
Practice council	Education and training	Meeting	Monthly
Service council	Customer service	Meeting	Monthly
Administration council	Hospital leadership	Meeting	Weekly
Clinical operations	Managers from all departments	Meeting	Monthly
One-on-one interviews	Personal perception of feedback	Interview	As needed
Nurses	Individual feedback	E-mail	As received

ask research questions 1 and 2 and record the responses. I will also conduct one-on-one interviews focused on these two research questions with the chief nursing officer of the hospital and the manager of the medical–surgical unit. In addition, the clinicians of the medical–surgical unit will be e-mailed an introduction to the study and then asked to respond to research questions 1 and 2 via e-mail.

The highlight of stage 2 is the introduction of the prototype audit and feedback report. At this point all staff members will receive a weekly e-mail explaining the purpose of the report, instructions on how to access it and submit suggestions for improvement and any other thoughts or questions they might have. The main objective during this stage is to identify barriers to accessing and understanding the report. I will continue to attend the five meetings and do one-on-one interviews with the chief nursing officer and the department manager. In this stage, I will start coming onto the nursing unit and answering questions from the staff about the report and obtaining their feedback for improvements or simply reflections on how well they like it or not. As each week passes, I will analyze the data on who is accessing the report or who is not. During the unit visits, I will target those who are viewing the data regularly as well as those who are not participating to collect their insights.

Stages 3 and 4 are considered revision stages. In the third stage I will follow the same approach to analysis as in the second but with a new version of the report containing changes as recommended by the co-researchers. The fourth stage will follow the same process as the third, except that this time I will reassess research questions 1 and 2 by asking the co-researchers to assess the questions using the EDW prototype process instead of the MDR review.

Data Analysis

Qualitative Analysis

Qualitative analysis will be the primary method used in this study. All research questions except question 5 will involve qualitative analysis. Most of the data will come from transcriptions of the digitally recorded meetings, interviews, field notes, e-mails, and surveys in each stage using two different coding cycles.

The first cycle will use both values coding and provisional coding as described by Saldaña (2009). Values coding focuses on understanding the participants' perspective, which is a summation of their values, attitudes, and beliefs (Saldaña, 2009). As noted in Chapter 2 of the dissertation, a major part of Bandura's (1991) self-regulation theory consists of judgmental and self-reactive processes, both of which are greatly influenced by a person's perspective (Bandura, 1991). The research questions include language that focuses on ascertaining the nurses' perceptions. For example, according to the nurses, what is the purpose of audit and feedback? What do nurses perceive about . . . ? In what ways, if any, do the audit and feedback processes influence them? What was collaboratively learned in creating the prototype audit and feedback? What are the nurses' opinions of the relative merits of . . . ? Analyses of the answers to these questions will build an understanding of the nurses' perspectives and lead to learning and identifying areas for improvement. Once these areas are identified, I can implement improvements in the process as suggested by the nurses.

Provisional coding, on the other hand, uses predefined codes that come from previous research studies, theories, investigator experience, or models; these are used as a starting point and can evolve or change over time (Saldaña, 2003). As already discussed, the purpose of this research is to explore whether audit and feedback designed using Bandura's (1991) system of self-regulation resonates positively with frontline nurses. Bandura's system involves seven concepts that are used here as predefined codes. Over the course of the study, each of these concepts, as represented in audit and feedback, will be evaluated for relevance and either changed, discarded, or improved. New concepts may be introduced as determined by the nurses. Provisional coding thus provides a way to ascertain whether or how Bandura's system of self-regulation is applicable to audit and feedback in this particular local context.

After the first cycle of coding (values and provisional) is completed, a second cycle will be used to reanalyze the data, looking for changes in the data between each stage. This second cycle will use longitudinal coding,

Table 4.9 *Longitudinal Coding Process*

Steps	Questions
Descriptive in-phase matrix	7 questions
Longitudinal cross-phase matrix comparison	6 questions

described by Saldaña (2009) as "appropriate for longitudinal qualitative studies that explore change and development in individuals, groups, and organization through extended periods of time" (2009, p. 176). It is thus well suited to measuring changes in nurses' perceptions of audit and feedback over time. The results, along with suggested changes made to the process, will also help determine the validity of rapid-cycle PAR research driven by frontline nurses for developing the prototype EDW audit and feedback process.

Saldaña (2009) has provided a template for beginning longitudinal research consisting of two distinct steps, each with specific questions as shown in Table 4.9. The longitudinal coding process that will be used in this study follows the outline created by Saldaña (2009, p. 174).

The first step of the longitudinal coding process is completed by answering seven questions that form the descriptive in-phase matrix (Saldaña, 2009, pp. 175–176), shown in Table 4.10. These questions identify types of changes over time within a phase. The answers to these questions then provide data for the second step of the analysis, which looks at various differences in the assessments from the first step across phases. The goal of these two steps is "to generate documented observations of meaningful human actions across time to extract processes (themes, trends, patterns, and so on)" (2003, pp. 64–65).

Table 4.10 *Descriptive In-Phase Matrix*

Questions

1. What increases or emerges through time?
2. What is cumulative through time?
3. What kinds of surges, epiphanies, or turning points occur through time?
4. What decreases or ceases through time?
5. What remains constant or consistent through time?
6. What is idiosyncratic through time?
7. What is missing through time?

Table 4.11 *Longitudinal Matrix Comparison Questions*

Questions

1. What are the differences between the descriptive matrices from previous phases?
2. What contextual or intervening conditions appear to influence participant changes through time?
3. What matrix interrelationships (cause and effect) exist through time?
4. Do the changes harmonize with or oppose what was expected based on Bandura's (1991) self-regulatory system and Edmondson and Schein's (2012) teaming theories?
5. Do the participants' changes follow any distinct rhythms?
6. What preliminary assertions can be deduced so far in this and previous phases?

An important element of this second (longitudinal) cycle of coding involves partitioning the data into distinct stages, as shown in Table 4.7. Each stage introduces a nuance that the previous stage did not have. An example of such a modification would be nurses starting to post in the break room a list of their names along with their performance in establishing a pain goal for everyone to see at the start of Stage 3. Each stage therefore goes through a descriptive analysis of changes over time.

The second step in the longitudinal coding cycle is known as the longitudinal phase matrix comparison. Whereas the first step involves analyzing changes within the study stage, the second step focuses on the differences between the current stage and the previous stage (Saldaña, 2009) as shown in Table 4.11. For example, the number of nurses accessing the audit and feedback in Stage 2 may suddenly increase over that in Stage 1.

Quantitative Analysis

Quantitative analysis will be carried out using McNemar's test with research questions 1 and 5. Research question 1 assesses how many nurses know the stated purpose of the MDR audit and feedback process and that of the EDW prototype. The nurses will be asked to respond to this question at the beginning of the study regarding the MDR process and, again, at the end regarding the prototype EDW process. Research question 5 compares the pain assessment documentation (Table 4.5) rate between the same 3-month period in 2012 and the study 3-month period in 2013.

A run chart will also be created showing how often the EDW prototype feedback report was accessed over the 3-month period. The run chart will help pinpoint which nurses are accessing the report and which are not, and this information will be used for follow-up interviews with the nurses.

Rigor of Action Research

Unlike positivist research, which can use the same concepts of rigor (e.g., reliability, external validity, internal validity, and generalizability) for evaluating the quality of the research, qualitative research involves several different concepts of rigor, some of which have been modified to meet the goals of this study. Herr and Anderson (2005, pp. 55) defined five concepts that together describe the goal and rigor of action research and are as follows: (a) Generation of new knowledge equates to dialogic and process validity; (b) achievement of action-oriented outcomes equates to dialogic and process validity; (c) education of both researcher and participants equates to catalytic validity; (d) results that are relevant to the local setting equate to democratic validity; (e) a sound and appropriate research methodology equates to process validity.

The goal of generating new knowledge establishes validity using dialogic and process validity. Dialogic validity involves having other researchers play the role of the devil's advocate in interpreting what other meanings could be derived from the results (Herr & Anderson, 2005). In this study, a reflection session will be held at the end of Stage 2 and before starting Stage 3 to obtain different viewpoints from outside experts and members of my dissertation committee vis-à-vis interpreting the results and making recommendations moving forward. Process validity for this goal will involve examining whether a problem has been presented accurately, while also promoting learning from co-researchers within the study (Herr & Anderson, 2005). Therefore, throughout this study I will conduct semistructured interviews with the co-researchers that will include questions such as what have they learned thus far. I will also keep an ongoing journal where I can reflect on what I am learning during the study. Both dialogic and process validity actions as planned will further support claims of generating new knowledge.

Outcome validity is synonymous with the term *integrity* (Herr & Anderson, 2005; Jacobson, 1998). Exploring and applying Bandura's (1991) theory of self-regulation and Edmondson and Schein's (2012) theory on teaming in designing the interventions of this study help support its integrity and subsequent outcomes. The theory-coding schema, as mentioned in the literature review, is used to further support outcome validity; the results of that analysis can be found in Appendix 4C. This schema meticulously analyzes the interaction and application of theory and how it is applied and measured within the research. Simply having successful outcomes from a study without due diligence to its overall planning, design, and execution do not meet the criteria for outcome validity.

Lather (1986) best described catalytic validity as "the degree to which the research process reorients, focuses, and energizes participants toward knowing reality in order to transform it. This is a process Freire (1973) terms conscientization" (p. 272). One reason the PAR methodology is a natural fit for this research lies in how it supports multiple cycles of improvements as well as catalytic validity. The researchers' perspectives on the value of audit and feedback and how well it helps them improve pain management over time will serve as the measure for catalytic validity. Another view of catalytic validity considers goals or purposes, as described by Herr and Anderson (2005); this involves the ongoing education of the researcher and participants (co-researchers) in finding solutions to problems.

Democratic validity guards against solving a problem without the participation of everyone with a stake in the problem. If such a scenario occurred, the solution would not meet the goal of democratic validity, which is to benefit all (Herr & Anderson, 2005). To ensure democratic validity in this study, all employees on the medical–surgical unit will be invited to share their perspectives by participating in unit meetings or via e-mail and periodic surveys.

Process validity also involves a cycle of examining the definition of the problem and the way it is framed, while questioning the assumptions behind it and how much is being learned about it (Herr & Anderson, 2005). It is measured by analyzing feedback given by co-researchers. Some good questions for the analysis in this study include: How many new ideas for modifying the audit and feedback are being given in each phase? How often is audit and feedback being accessed in each phase? What were the initial perceptions of co-researchers about pain management, and how have those perceptions changed over time? If during the study there is a decrease in feedback or the feedback is not being accessed as frequently, this would indicate potential process validity issues.

Process validity in this study will be measured by a longitudinal analysis of the data, which will facilitate validity by comparing the differences in answers to the above questions and others between the phases of the study. One of the many benefits of having multiple ways of receiving feedback from the co-researchers will be keeping a pulse on process validity.

Limitations

This research is focused on developing audit and feedback for one clinical issue (acute pain management) on one nursing unit in one hospital over a relatively short time. Although the final audit and feedback report developed for showing compliance to charting required pain assessments when giving an opioid medication at this one hospital cannot be expected to work at all hospitals, the process of developing the report will be generalizable.

Conflicts about the value of PAR may be perceived as a limitation in producing generalizable knowledge for other practice situations. Herr and Anderson (2005) described two opposing views of action research in other fields (e.g., education) between academics (outsiders) and practitioners (insiders). Academics claim that although action research may be applied to a current practice, it cannot be generalized as public knowledge with epistemic claims. Practitioners, on the other hand, believe that academic research is void of understanding (a) the practitioner's real-life challenges, such as settings, relationships, and subjective reality, and (b) the ways in which practitioners (insiders) work together in PAR, where both strengths and views are brought together in generating new knowledge.

Anticipated Barriers and Challenges

One potential challenge in this study is obtaining the participation of the approximately 40 frontline nurses who work on the medical–surgical unit. It is unknown how much of their participation I will be able to elicit, especially because I do not work in either the unit or the hospital and so am classified as an outsider. I will nonetheless try to elicit feedback from each one through various meetings, surveys, site visits, and e-mails. In my favor I have the support of the chief nursing officer and the nurse unit manager, who will assist me in better connecting with the nurses. In addition, the nursing unit has established a goal this year to achieve 90% pain documentation.

Because I am both the PI and an outsider, I will need to listen to the nurses and identify and address any barriers that may prevent me from working with them effectively. Some nurses may develop ill feelings toward me for having their performance data posted in the nursing unit for staff to view. It is therefore essential that the nurses feel that the decisions made during the study are their own and not being imposed upon them by me. To mitigate this situation, I will have frequent, open communications with all nurses and hospital management and address any issues that may arise.

The hospital's recent citation by The Joint Commission for failing to chart the reassessment of the PIS per protocol may improve the compliance to charting the PIS prior to starting the study. Hospitals routinely go through a Joint Commission review, and when they receive a direct finding, they are required to submit a plan to the commission and achieve 90% compliance over a 3-month period. In this case, the period happened to fall at the end of

2012. Although additional attention is being given to reassessing pain interventions with the goal of improving compliance, understanding the impact of The Joint Commission is valuable because its reviews commonly occur in all hospitals. This will also provide an opportunity to see what will happen with compliance performance over time once The Joint Commission trial period has ended. Nonetheless, The Joint Commission finding at the hospital under study also creates a perceived barrier in that this history will alter the outcomes and so pose a threat to the study's internal validity.

Finally, it is very likely that suggestions for changing current hospital pain protocols or EMR pain charting will be made, but changes made to either pain protocols or electronic charting may take longer than this study will last. Every effort will be made to expedite these changes if they are requested, but they are not required for the study to be completed. In addition, changes to the audit and feedback report may take longer than expected when requested, although the personnel needed (data architects and business intelligence developers) to make future changes are already planning on these changes with the expectation or hope of delivering on requests as soon as possible.

REFERENCES

Ajzen, I. (1991). The theory of planned behavior. *Organizational Behavior and Human Decision Processes, 50*(2), 179–211.

Archibald, L. H., Ott, M. J., Gale, C. M., Zhang, J., Peters, M. S., & Stroud, G. K. (2011). Enhanced recovery after colon surgery in a community hospital system. *Diseases of the Colon & Rectum, 54*(7), 840–845.

Argyris, C., & Schon, D. (1989). Participatory action research and action science compared. *American Behavioral Scientist, 32*(5), 612–623.

Baker, R., Camosso-Stefinovic, J., Gillies, C., Shaw, E. J., Cheater, F., Flottorp, S., & Robertson, N. (2010). Tailored interventions to overcome identified barriers to change: Effects on professional practice and health care outcomes. *Cochrane Database of Systematic Reviews, 2010*(3). doi:10.1002/14651858.CD005470.pub2 Retrieved from http://www.mrw.interscience.wiley.com/cochrane/clsysrev/articles/CD005470/frame.html

Bandura, A. (1991). Social cognitive theory of self-regulation. *Organizational Behavior and Human Decision Processes, 50*(2), 248–287. doi:10.1016/0749-5978(91)90022-l

Bandura, A. (1997). *Self-efficacy: The exercise of control.* New York, NY: Freeman.

Clarke, D. D. (1987). Fundamental problems with fundamental research: A meta–theory for social psychology. *Philosophica, 40*, 23–61.

Committee on the Robert Wood Johnson Foundation Initiative on the Future of Nursing, at the Institute of Medicine. (2011). *The future of nursing: Leading change, advancing health.* Washington, DC: National Academies Press.

Drach-Zahavy, A., & Pud, D. (2010). Learning mechanisms to limit medication administration errors. *Journal of Advanced Nursing, 66*(4), 794–805. doi:10.1111/j.1365-2648.2010.05294.x

Edmondson, A. C. (2002). The local and variegated nature of learning in organizations: A group-level perspective. *Organization Science, 13*(2), 128–146.

Edmondson, A. C., & Schein, E. H. (2012). *Teaming: How organizations learn, innovate, and compete in the knowledge economy.* San Franscisco, CA: Jossey-Bass.

Foy, R., Eccles, M. P., Jamtvedt, G., Young, J., Grimshaw, J. M., & Baker, R. (2005). What do we know about how to do audit and feedback? Pitfalls in applying evidence from a systematic review. *BMC Health Services Research, 5,* 50–57. doi:10.1186/1472-6963-5-50

Freire, P. (1973). *Pedagogy of the oppressed.* New York, NY: Seabury Press.

Greenhalgh, T., Robert, G., Macfarlane, F., Bate, P., & Kyriakidou, O. (2004). Diffusion of innovations in service organizations: Systematic review and recommendations. *Milbank Quarterly, 82*(4), 581–629. doi:10.1111/j.0887-378X.2004.00325.x

Grimshaw, J. M., Thomas, R. E., MacLennan, G., Fraser, C., Ramsay, C. R., Vale, L., . . . Donaldson, C. (2004). Effectiveness and efficiency of guideline dissemination and implementation strategies. *Health Technology Assessment, 8*(6), iii–iv, 1–72.

Grol, R. P. T. M., Bosch, M. C., Hulscher, M. E. J. L., Eccles, M. P., & Wensing, M. (2007). Planning and studying improvement in patient care: The use of theoretical perspectives. *Milbank Quarterly, 85*(1), 93–138. doi:10.1111/j.1468-0009.2007.00478.x

Hammermeister, K. (2009). The National Surgical Quality Improvement Program: Learning from the past and moving to the future. *American Journal of Surgery, 198*(5 Suppl), S69–S73.

Harvard Business School. (2012). Faculty & research. Retrieved November 17, 2012 from http://www.hbs.edu/faculty/Pages/profile.aspx?facId=6451

Hayes, R., Bratzler, D., Armour, B., Moore, L., Murray, C., Stevens, B. R., . . . Ballard, D. J. (2001). Comparison of an enhanced versus a written feedback model on the management of Medicare inpatients with venous thrombosis. *Joint Commission Journal on Quality Improvement, 27*(3), 155–168.

Herr, K., & Anderson, G. L. (2005). *The action research dissertation: A guide for students and faculty.* Thousand Oaks, CA: Sage Publications, Inc.

Hillman, A. L., & Ripley, K. (1999). The use of physician financial incentives and feedback to improve pediatric preventive care in medicine. *Pediatrics, 104*(4), 931.

Hughes, R. (2008). *Patient safety and quality: An evidence-based handbook for nurses.* Rockville, MD: United States Agency for Healthcare Research and Quality.

Illionois Hospital Association. (2011). Value-based purchasing: Questions and answers. Retrieved March 8, 2011, from www.ihatoday.org/uploadDocs/1/vbpurch.pdf

Ingraham, A. M., Richards, K. E., Hall, B. L., & Ko, C. Y. (2010). Quality improvement in surgery: The American College of Surgeons National Surgical Quality Improvement Program approach. *Advances In Surgery, 44,* 251–267.

Ivers, N., Jamtvedt, G., Flottorp, S., Young, J. M., Odgaard-Jensen, J., French, S. D., . . . Oxman, A. D. (2012). Audit and feedback: Effects on professional practice and healthcare outcomes. *Cochrane Database of Systematic Reviews (Online), 2012*(6), CD000259.

Jacobson, W. (1998). Defining the quality of practitioner research. *Adult Education Quarterly, 48*(3), 125.

Jamtvedt, G., Young, J. M., Kristoffersen, D. T., O'Brien, M. A., & Oxman, A. D. (2006). Audit and feedback: Effects on professional practice and health care outcomes. *Cochrane Database of Systematic Reviews, 2006*(2). doi:10.1002/14651858.CD000259. pub2   Retrieved   from   http://www.mrw.interscience.wiley.com/cochrane /clsysrev/articles/CD000259/frame.html

Kelley, K., Bond, R., & Abraham, C. (2001). Effective approaches to persuading pregnant women to quit smoking: A meta-analysis of intervention evaluation studies. *British Journal of Health Psychology, 6*(3), 207.

Kluger, A. N., & DeNisi, A. (1996). The effects of feedback interventions on performance. *Psychological Bulletin, 119*(2), 254.

Kohn, L. T., Corrigan, J., & Donaldson, M. S. (2000). *To Err Is Human: Building a Safer Health System.* Washington, DC: National Academies Press.

Kohn, L. T., Corrigan, J. M., & Donaldson, M. S. (2001). *Crossing the quality chasm: A new health system for the 21st century.* Washington, DC: Committee on Quality of Health Care in America, Institute of Medicine.

Lather, P. (1986). Research as praxis. *Harvard Educational Review, 56,* 257–277.

Meyer, J. (2000). Qualitative research in health care. Using qualitative methods in health related action research. *BMJ (Clinical Research Ed.), 320*(7228), 178–181.

Michie, S, & Abraham, C. (2004). Interventions to change health behaviours: Evidence-based or evidence-inspired? *Psychology & Health, 19*(1), 29–49.

Michie, J., Francis, H., & Eccles, M. (2008). From theory to intervention: Mapping theoretically derived behavioural determinants to behaviour change techniques. *Applied Psychology: An International Review, 57*(4), 660–680. doi:10.1111/j.1464-0597.2008.00341.x

Michie, S., & Prestwich, A. (2010). Are interventions theory-based? Development of a theory coding scheme. *Health Psychology, 29*(1), 1–8. doi:10.1037/a0016939

Michie, S., Webb, T. L., & Sniehotta, F. F. (2010). The importance of making explicit links between theoretical constructs and behaviour change techniques. *Addiction, 105*(11), 1897–1898.

Needleman, J., Kurtzman, E. T., & Kizer, K. W. (2007). Performance measurement of nursing care: State of the science and the current consensus. *Medical Care Research & Review, 64*(2), 10S–43S.

Needleman, J., Pearson, M., Parkerton, P., Uneniek, V., Soban, L., Bakas, A., & Yee, T. (2007). *Tranforming care at the bedside: Lessons from Phase II—Executive summary.* Los Angeles, CA: UCLA.

Parker, L. E., de Pillis, E., Altschuler, A., Rubenstein, L. V., & Meredith, L. S. (2007). Balancing participation and expertise: A comparison of locally and centrally managed health care quality improvement within primary care practices. *Qualitative Health Research, 17*(9), 1268–1279.

Parkerton, P. H., Needleman, J., Pearson, M. L., Upenieks, V. V., Soban, L. M., & Yee, T. (2009). Lessons from nursing leaders on implementing TCAB: Feedback from chief nursing officers and unit managers. *American Journal of Nursing, 109*(11), 71–76. doi:10.1097/01.naj.0000362030.08494.22

Saldaña, J. (2003). *Longitudinal qualitative research: Analyzing change through time.* Walnut Creek, CA: AltaMira Press.

Saldaña, J. (2009). *The coding manual for qualitative researchers.* Thousand Oaks, CA: Sage.

Sauaia, A., Ralston, D., Schluter, W. W., Marciniak, T. A., Havranek, E. P., & Dunn, T. R. (2000). Influencing care in acute myocardial infarction: A randomized trial comparing 2 types of intervention. *American Journal Of Medical Quality: The Official Journal Of The American College Of Medical Quality, 15*(5), 197–206.

Tucker, A. L., & Edmondson, A. C. (2003). Why hospitals don't learn from failures: Organizational and psychological dynamics that inhibit system change. *California Management Review, 45*(2), 55–72.

APPENDIX 4A

Baker 2003

Aim: Determine if the format of guidelines determines adoption for management of asthma and angina

Theory: Not mentioned

Interventions:

1. Full evidence-based guidelines
2. Prioritized review evidence-based guidelines (peer reviewed and summarized)
3. Prioritized review with feedback

Ferguson 2003

Aim: Determine if low intensity continuous quality improvement (CQI) interventions increases adoption rate

Theory: Not mentioned

Interventions:

1. No intervention material
2. Perioperative blockade, local opinion leader, call to action letter, feedback, plan, slide set, contact info
3. Internal mammary artery (IMA) grafting, local opinion leader, call to action letter, feedback, plan, slide set, contact info

Goff 2003

Aim: Determine if mailing guideline summaries, peer comparison feedback, and chart reminders increases therapies to mortality rates of persons with congestive heart disease

Theory: Yes

Interventions:

1. Control condition
2. Mailed American Heart Association (AHA) guidelines, peer comparison feedback, patient specific chart reminders

Hayes 2001

Aim: Improved anticoagulation management

Theory: Yes

Interventions:

1. Mailed guidelines, feedback, data collection tool, quality improvement (QI) plan, references
2. Control group material plus meetings with CQI physician and project liaison, slide show, video

Hendryx 1998

Aim: Rural hospital improvement of patient (ventilated) care processes, patient mortality and morbidity, resource use

Theory: Not mentioned

Interventions:

1. Control group
2. Outreach program, physicians, nurses, respiratory therapist, dieticians, with telephone follow-up

Hillman 1999

Research Question: A system of semiannual assessment and feedback increases pediatric preventive care

Theory: Not mentioned

Interventions:

1. Control group
2. Physicians received mailed written feedback on compliance
3. Physicians received mailed written feedback on compliance plus financial bonus

Katz 2004

Research question: Improve compliance to smoking guideline as recommended in primary care settings

Theory: Not mentioned

Interventions:

1. Agency for Healthcare Research & Quality (AHRQ) guidelines
2. AHRQ guidelines plus tutorial intake clinicians plus individual and group feedback

Kerse 1999

Research question: Establish effect of education intervention for general practitioners on elderly patients

Theory: Not mentioned

Interventions:

1. Control group
2. Educational program and clinical practice audit

Kinsinger 1998

Research question: Performance rates of breast cancer screening

Theory: Not mentioned

Interventions:

1. Control group
2. Meetings with MD investigators with practice physicians and staff plus feedback plus suggestions for improvement

Lemelin 1998

Aim: Prevention facilitation in primary care

Theory: Not mentioned

Interventions:

1. Control group
2. Multifaceted intervention with nurse facilitator

Leviton 1999

Aim: Appropriate us of antenatal corticosteroids

Theory: Not mentioned

Interventions:

1. Usual dissemination of practice recommendations
2. Usual dissemination plus focused dissemination effort

Lomas 1993

Research question: Appropriate use of cesarean section

Theory: Not mentioned

Interventions:

1. Passive dissemination of guidelines
2. Guidelines plus education via opinion leader
3. Guidelines plus audit and feedback

Manfredi 1998

Research question: Evaluate HMO intervention to increase cancer screenings in primary care

Theory: Not mentioned

Interventions:

1. Mailed letter from Chicago HMO endorsing National Cancer Institute (NCI) guidelines
2. Onsite training, start up assistance, MD education, QA visits, plus MD feedback

O'Connell 2003

Research question: Increase prescribing of lower cost generic drugs than newer more expensive drugs

Theory: Not mentioned

Interventions:

1. No information on prescribing practices
2. Mailed individual feedback with graphs of prescribing rates plus educational newsletters

Primlott 2003

Research question: Reduction of benzodiazepine prescriptions

Theory: Not mentioned

Interventions:

1. Mailed feedback and educational bulletins about first-line antihypertension
2. Mailed Benzo prescribing practice plus educational bulletin

Quinley 2004

Research question: Improved office based adult immunization

Theory: Not mentioned

Interventions:

1. Mailed letter showing that their coverage rate of pneumococcal polysaccharide vaccine (PPV) was lower than average
2. Control plus follow-up phone call

Sauaia 2000

Research question: Improving acute myocardial infarction care

Theory: Not mentioned

Interventions:

1. Mailed feedback
2. On-site presentation to evaluate performance feedback

Sondergaard 2002

Research question: Improved usage of asthma drugs

Theory: Not mentioned

Interventions:

1. Mailed feedback on unrelated subject
2. Mailed patient-specific data on asthma drug prescribing patterns and guidelines

Sondergaard 2003

Research question: Improved antibiotics prescribing

Theory: Not mentioned

Interventions:

1. Mailed guidelines on antibiotics
2. Mailed clinical guidelines and aggregated data on prescribing antibiotics

Soumerai 1998

Research Question: Improved thrombolytics, beta-blockers, decrease prophylactic lidocaine

Theory: Not mentioned

Interventions:

1. Mailed data feedback on study drugs to medical director
2. Opinion leaders held group discussions about drug efficacy, comparative performance, and barriers to change

Thompson 2000

Research question: Increased asking about and treating domestic violence in primary care

Theory: Yes

Interventions:

1. Control group
2. Training sessions, bimonthly newsletter, clinical education rounds, feedback, posters

Verstappen 2003

Research question: Improved primary care test ordering

Theory: Not mentioned

Interventions:

1. ARM A cardiovascular topics
2. ARM B chronic obstructive pulmonary disease (COPD), asthma, degenerative joint complaints

Vingerhoets 2001

Research question: Improved care of primary care patients from patients' perspectives

Theory: Not mentioned

Interventions:

1. Control group
2. Individualized structured feedback based on patient ratings

Wells 2000

Research question: If quality improvement (QI) programs in managed care practice improve care, health outcomes, and employment of depressed patients

Theory: Not mentioned

Interventions:

1. Mailed AHRQ guidelines for depression
2. QI-Meds (RN follow-up). Train local experts, lectures, academic detailing, audit and feedback, extra resources (staff)
3. QI-Therapy (Therapist). Train local experts, lectures, academic detailing, audit and feedback, extra staff resources

---

APPENDIX 4B

Example of Feedback for Reassessing Pain After Interventions

Accuracy: Nurses know they are being monitored and are able to validate dates (by clicking on the account numbers of specific patients).

Performance Attribution: Nurses attribute personal efforts to the goal (see the name next to the intervention and whether the reassessment was met or not or how efforts helped the unit overall).

Referential Performance: Nurses see the performance of their unit/hospital in relation to others.

Informativeness: Nurses see personal progress toward goal.

Nurse	Patient Reassessment Opportunities	Reassessment Completed	Reassessment Rate/Goal	Unit Reassessment Opportunities	Unit Reassessments	Attribution to Total Patients Reassessed on Unit (Actual/ Max)
Nurse A	30	18	60%/90%	300	250	7%/12%

Medicare Hospital Compare Patient Survey Question

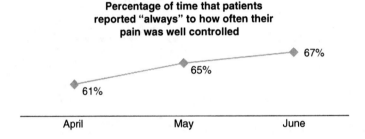

Percentage of time that patients reported "always" to how often their pain was well controlled

61% 65% 67%

April   May   June

Valuation: Nurses can see that doing pain reassessment within an hour of the intervention benefits the patient, and so they will value this behavioral more and be more compliant.

Regularity: Nurses receive weekly e-mails with a link and reminder that the report is updated daily and can be accessed at any time.

Temporal Proximity

1. The main measurement is taken on whether the pain reassessment was completed within 60 minutes of the pain intervention, not on how well patients rated their pain as under control. Compliance with performing the pain intervention within an hour is more proximate than the patients' overall rating.
2. Charting data from that day will be available within 24 hours on the report. The report is proximate to the time of charting.

APPENDIX 4C

Overview of Theory-Coding Scheme

Category 1: Is theory mentioned?

Item no.	Item	Yes/no/ don't know	List with location in paper
1	Theory of behavioral mentioned	Yes	Self-regulation, p. XX
2	Targeted construct mentioned as predictor of behavioral	Yes	Self-regulation, p. XX Teaming, p. XX
3	Intervention based on single theory	Yes	Self-regulation, p. XX

Category 1 looks for any evidence that a behavioral theory is used, and then for specifics about the targeted construct and whether the intervention is based on a single theory. All three items in this category are accounted for with page references. Edmondson and Schein's (2012) construct of teaming is not a theory like Bandura's (1991) self-regulation theory but rather is a construct that predicts behavioral.

Category 2: Are the relevant theoretical constructs targeted?

Item no.	Item	Yes/no/ don't know	List with location in paper
2	Targeted construct mentioned as predictor of behavioral	Yes	Self-regulation, p. XX Teaming, p. XX
5	Theory/predicators used to select/develop intervention technique	Yes	EDW feedback, p. XX
7	All intervention techniques explicitly linked to at least one theory-relevant construct/ predictor	Yes	EDW feedback, p. XX

Category 2 specifies whether the targeted constructs are mentioned, then determines if they were used in designing the intervention and if all interventions are linked to the constructs. Category 2 is confirmatory if the theory and targeted constructs really are used in the overall design of all interventions.

Category 3: Is theory used to select recipients or tailor interventions?

Item no.	Item	Yes/no/ don't know	List with location in paper
4	Theory/predictors used to select recipients for the intervention	No	Based on methodology, p. XX
6	Theory/predictors used to tailor intervention techniques to recipients	Yes	Integrated learning, p. XX

Category 3 involves selecting the best recipients for the interventions and describing how the theory or predictors are customized for them. No pretests were given to determine whether the clinicians on the medical–surgical unit were the best fit for this intervention; rather, the unit was chosen because of the local problem of needing to improve the management of their pain care. Not only are the interventions used for this study tailored for the medical–surgical clinicians, but the clinicians, in turn, also determine how best to modify the interventions to help them in managing their patients' pain.

Category 4: Are the relevant theoretical concepts measured?

Item no.	Item	Yes/no/ don't know	List with location in paper
12	Theory-relevant constructs/ predictors are measured b. At least one construct of theory (or predictor) mentioned in relation to the intervention is measured pre- and postintervention	b. Yes	Research questions, p. XX
13	Quality of measures b. All measures of theory-relevant constructs/predictors had some evidence of reliability c. All measures of theory-relevant constructs/predictors have been previously validated d. Behavioral measures had some evidence for their reliability e. Behavioral measure has been previously validated f. Behavior measure has been previously validated	b. Yes d. Yes e. Yes f. Yes	Rigor of action research, p. XX

Category 4 looks for measurements of Bandura's (1991) self-regulating theory and Edmondson and Schein's (2012) concept of teaming in the study and evidence of reliability and validity in those measures.

Category 5: Is theory tested?

Item no.	Item	Yes/no/ don't know	List with location in paper
14	Randomization of participants to condition	No	Based on methodology, p. XX
15	Changes in measured theory-relevant constructs/predictor	TBD	
16	Mediational analysis of construct(s)/ predictor(s)	TBD	
17	Results discussed in relation to theory	TBD	
18	Appropriate support for theory	TBD	

TBD, to be determined.

Category 5 looks at the quality of randomization, outcomes, and mediational analysis, and at how the results are tied back to the theory and constructs. Randomization was not necessary for this study, and the participants were selected based on the methodology. The remaining items will be determined during the analysis of the data. No mediational analysis is done in this research but rather a qualitative analysis accompanied by a couple of simple quantitative metrics. This is a change from the original theory-coding schema (Michie & Prestwich, 2010) with modifications made for this study.

Category 6: Are results used to refine theory?

Item No.	Item	Yes/no/ don't know	List with location in paper
19	Results used to refine theory	TBD	

TBD, to be determined.

COMMENTARY TO "WHEN DESCRIPTION IS NOT ENOUGH: ACTION AS PARTICIPATORY RESEARCH"

Lauren Clark

In qualitative methods, PAR stands apart. It tells us that description is not enough and that action is the currency of social change, the public good born of research. In nursing and the health sciences we see PAR conducted in communities, notably in inner cities, on reservations, with older adults, and in scores of other communities around the world. By partnering with the participants in research, investigators share with them the goal of arriving at actionable research outcomes. And in the process of participating in research, they learn together (Flaskerud & Anderson, 1999).

PAR and related research approaches are not a method, per se, but an orientation to research that engages community members and researchers in a cooperative endeavor, achieves a balance of research and action, and develops community capacity while empowering participants to increase control over their lives (Israel, Schulz, Parker, & Becker, 1998; Minkler & Wallerstein, 2008). Action-oriented research approaches have been widely used with a variety of vulnerable populations because they remain "the most viable attempt to respect community autonomy in public health research today" (Buchanan, Miller, & Wallerstein, 2007).

The range of participation in PAR varies, from forming an advisory board that convenes periodically to advise the research team, to coding, interpreting, and publishing the research as co-equal participants. As Matthew Peters points out in his study of nurses' attention to patient pain, PAR changes both the responsibilities of the researcher and the participants. Depending on the purpose, epistemology, ideological commitments, disciplinary background, and research traditions of the researcher, PAR has close cousins that share similar tenets. These include action research, collaborative inquiry, feminist action research, emancipatory practice, community-engaged research, and community-based participatory research (Herr & Anderson, 2005). Cycles of action characterize this sort of research and the period after research.

Working with the participants or the community, rather than on it, holds promise. Recalcitrant clinical care problems have remained in the face of policies, checklists, incentives, and, most recently, withholding pay to hospitals or providers for substandard care. Complex health care organizations need research to help protect patients from mistakes and ensure high quality care. To explore more fully how and why nurses might consider action research, I held a discussion with students in a graduate-level qualitative research course. What are the reasons that participatory and action research is gaining interest and popularity in the health sciences at this moment in time? Below are our reflections.

REASONS TO CONSIDER PAR AND OTHER PARTICIPATORY RESEARCH APPROACHES

1. It's the right time. Many communities complain of being "studied to death." They are ready for us to make good on promises to help lead change through research.
2. Suspicion of research can be overcome. Historical specters of breaches in research ethics with poor or marginalized groups means we need more accountability for their ethical involvement in research.
3. The results of engaged research are meaningful at the local level because they are produced at the local level. The town/gown divide between communities and universities can be addressed if we focus on local problems near us with the involvement of our neighbors.
4. Whole-person or whole-community research is needed to balance sub-cellular basic science research. There is space and value for both kinds of science.
5. It's an opportunity to work on justice and equity. We acknowledge the political aspect of our science when we explain that research is participatory and can lead action.

Finally, PAR is practical. It appeals to scientists who consider problems holistically, and offers a new approach to generating nursing science (Young, 2013).

REFERENCES

Buchanan, D. R., Miller, F. G., & Wallerstein, N. (2007). Ethical issues in community-based participatory research: Balancing rigorous research with community participation in community intervention studies. *Progress in Community Health Partnerships: Research, Education, and Action, 1,* 153–160.

Flaskerud, J. H., & Anderson, N. (1999). Disseminating the results of participant-focused research. *Journal of Transcultural Nursing, 10,* 340–349.

Israel, B. A., Schulz, A. J., Parker, E. A., & Becker, A. B. (1998). Review of community-based research: Assessing partnership approaches to improve public health. *Annual Reviews in Public Health, 19,* 73–202.

Minkler, M., & Wallerstein, N. (Eds.) (2008). *Community based participatory research for health: from process to outcomes* (2nd ed). San Francisco, CA: Jossey-Bass.

Young, L. E. (2013). Participatory action research: A new science for nursing? In C. T. Beck (Ed.), *Routledge international handbook of qualitative nursing research* (pp. 319–330). London, England: Routledge.

CHAPTER FIVE

COMMUNITY-BASED PARTICIPATORY RESEARCH IN THE DOMINICAN REPUBLIC: THE ON-THE-GROUND STORY OF CONDUCTING INTERNATIONAL PARTICIPATORY RESEARCH

Jennifer Foster

From 2008 to 2011, I was the principal investigator (PI) of a community-based participatory research (CBPR) study in the Dominican Republic, supported by the National Institute of Nursing Research in the United States. This chapter describes the study and my navigation of conducting cross-cultural research in a foreign country, but in a personal and pragmatic way, unlike the research reports previously published (Foster et al., 2010a, b; Foster et al., 2012).

The purpose of this chapter is to help other researchers who do CBPR or who want to do CBPR learn from both the successes and the mistakes of this project. No matter what anyone says, I believe conducting research is the best means to learn how to do research. All the best texts, journal articles, classes, or lectures cannot help you learn as much as actually doing research because there are so many nuances and decisions to make along the way. One strategizes the best one can, asks for advice from seasoned researchers, and learns by doing. One also has to accept that mistakes are inevitable, so it is best to accept that and learn from them. CBPR, by definition, is especially challenging because there are so many people with competing interests involved, and the outcomes are unpredictable. This CBPR study was especially challenging for a variety of reasons, including, but not limited to, the following: It was my first externally funded research study; it was an international, cross-cultural project; and we conducted it and analyzed it in Spanish (not my primary language).

To understand how this study came about, readers should know that as an academic nurse–midwife/anthropologist researcher, I made a commitment to CBPR as the approach of my research program for the duration of my career. However, I did not make this decision until after the completion of my dissertation in cultural anthropology. I say this because it is not in any doctoral student's best interest to do CBPR for their dissertation—it takes too long, and the research process is not always in the PI's control. Thus, a doctoral student conducting a CBPR study for the dissertation might not get out of graduate school for many years! Also, CBPR is not for everyone. Not everyone has the temperament suited to CBPR (Israel et al., 2008).

My personal commitment to CBPR did not develop until after I came to know the participants in my dissertation study. My dissertation was not participatory research; rather, it was an ethnographic study of Puerto Rican partners of adolescent mothers and how they constructed their masculine identity as fathers (Foster, 2004). The setting was a low-income, urban neighborhood in the United States, a place where I had worked as a nurse–midwife for a decade, caring for Puerto Rican adolescent mothers. When I began my field work in anthropology, I was worried that I, a White, middle-aged, female nurse–midwife, would have difficulty in gaining the trust of Puerto Rican, young males for meaningful interviews. Although it was difficult to recruit these men at first, once I had recruited them, they wanted to talk for hours. In fact, many of them were longing to talk to me about their experience of being a father. They felt the world outside their neighborhood perceived them as deadbeats, dropouts, drug addicts, and criminals, but never as fathers. They had a lot to say, and they wanted what they said disseminated far and wide; that is, they wanted their expert knowledge of their own condition to bear on all the discursive debates about adolescent single motherhood and fatherhood in the United States.

My dissertation study led me to realize that, if disparities in health are to be eliminated, their deconstruction is going to be made by the people affected by them—not by researchers coming in from the outside. This was quite an epiphany for a soon-to-be academic interested in health disparities research, who had devoted many years to doctoral research training. Nevertheless, the realization led to my understanding that CBPR is an approach, a different paradigm, of collaborative knowledge production, an intellectual space where academics can and do support the generation of community knowledge. Thus, I decided CBPR would be my approach to research wherever I would go in the future. This clarity has been very helpful in my journey as an academic; it is my moral compass, my true north. I lay this out for readers considering CBPR because it is easier to do traditional research and more advantageous for promotion and tenure, as CBPR publications take a long time and funding can be even more uncertain in an already tight funding environment. So, a novice researcher should be clear whether he or she is suited to CBPR and really wants to commit to it.

At the time of this writing, I have had opportunities to do CBPR in three different geographical locations. This chapter focuses on only one location, the project in the Dominican Republic because the CBPR in that setting has been the most developed and widely disseminated (probably because it had more funding than the other sites).

In 2004, I had the opportunity to become involved in a nascent partnership between U.S. nurse–midwives and nurses in the Dominican Republic, called the ADAMES Association. The ADAMES association is a nonprofit organization, managed by the International Agency of Charity, Dominican Chapter. The purpose of the organization is to improve maternal health and decrease maternal mortality in the San Francisco de Macoris setting of the Dominican Republic. A group of Dominican nurses, under the strong leadership of their nursing director, was concerned about maternal mortality in their hospital. They invited a consultation from U.S. nurse–midwives via the World Health Organization (WHO) collaborating centers system. The consultation, by mutual agreement, resulted in an educational project. For a few years, the project focused on educational conferences with the Dominican maternity nurses and two small, internally funded research studies our team conducted with the nurses as study participants (Foster, Burgos, Regueira, & Sanchez, 2005; Foster, Regueira, & Heath, 2006). As I got to know the nurses in the Dominican setting better over time, I realized this setting had great potential to do CBPR with possibilities for significant and positive nurse–community impact.

DESCRIPTION OF THE STUDY

CBPR requires time up front to develop relationships and trust within a community. Once that trust is established, various community members feel free to express some of their pressing questions, questions that research can answer. When the group of Dominican nurses asked why pregnant women delayed arrival at the maternity ward and came in such a deteriorated condition that the hospital was challenged to save them, I recognized the significance of the research question for both local and global health care professionals. So that became the research question for our study. The conceptual framework that we used for the study was the midwifery model of care, because that was the model that organized the entire ADAMES Association.

The midwifery model of care contains three concurrent process elements summarized as: provision of care that is woman-centered and humane, that applies evidence-based practices, and that incorporates the public health nursing intervention of case management and follow-up within the context of an interdisciplinary health care team (Foster & Heath, 2007). Only later did I realize how much the research question feeds into the wider framework of the four delay model, initially articulated by Thaddeus and Maine in 1994, but widely used around the world to explain the root causes of maternal mortality (Thaddeus & Maine, 1994).

The idea for the design of the study was an outcome of an observation by the United States midwives who had participated over the years (2004–2007) in the educational partnership. In general, providers felt blamed in the hospital when there was a maternal death. Maternal death is such a tragedy, not just for families, but for communities and even for nations (Sachs, 2005), that it is common for people to want to blame someone or some group. The community tended to blame the health providers for not giving good medical and nursing care, not valuing them as patients, and for not listening to their concerns. The health providers tended to blame the community for their lack of knowledge and for their lack of compliance with medical directives. Each group blamed the other.

To answer the research question that the nurses posed, it was clear to me, as a cultural anthropologist, that both groups needed to really hear each other's experiences. To listen to each other, they needed to work together and they both needed to hear the same information. This then launched the work of anthropology to explain how different groups can hear the same information but interpret it so differently. We needed to put nurses and community workers together, as one team, and discover, in a systematic and documented way, what the community knew and believed as they accessed publicly funded obstetrical care.

Hence, the study's aims were:

1. To orient and train a Dominican community-based team in CBPR in which team members were drawn from two different constituencies that share the common interest of improving the quality of obstetric care: lay community health workers (CHWs) represented one constituency, maternity health care personnel from the public hospital that served the neighborhoods where the CHWs reside represented the other constituency
2. To identify the relevant cultural knowledge, attitudes, beliefs, and behaviorals of pregnant and parous women as well as those of the male family members who have experienced maternal loss, which affect how women accessed and participated in publicly funded obstetrical care

3. To compare the differences between the interpretations of qualitative data analyzed by CHWs from the interpretations of qualitative data derived by maternity health care personnel and to build upon knowledge of the community's role in data analysis in CBPR.

The design was a three-phased, qualitative descriptive study, with each phase corresponding to each aim. In many ways, this project lent itself to an ethnographic approach because we had a long history of being present in the cultural milieu, and we used a variety of qualitative methods, including recorded field notes and memos, 12 focus groups, 12 semistructured interviews, and participant observations of 15 women followed prospectively for their prenatal care. Additionally, we audiotaped dialogues among research team members during the monthly meetings in Phase II and, at the time of analysis, in Phase III. The purpose of these recorded dialogues were, in part, to provide an audit trail about our process of data collection and analysis and, in part, to document differences in interpretations of data between CHWs and health providers.

We did not claim to use an ethnographic design, however, because I, as PI, was only able to be physically present in the Dominican Republic for 1- to 2-week periods of time, and I did not want to make a claim about the qualitative approach that some grant reviewers might question. Simply, a qualitative descriptive study felt a safer claim, and the acceptability of the value of this approach has been affirmed in the qualitative methodological literature (Sandelowski, 2000).

Phase I included training and orientation of the community-based research team. Anytime one does CBPR, one is confronted by structural power differences, and our work is to acknowledge them and constantly try and level them. As a U.S. PI with a PhD, I was in a more powerful position than the Dominican nurses, de facto. In turn, the Dominican nurses had a more powerful socioeconomic position than the community members. Consistently leveling these power differences was the single biggest challenge of this research. These power differences played out in every phase of the research. In the following section, I discuss how I handled the navigation of leveling these power differences in each of the project phases in turn.

The Dominican nurses had been involved in the planning of the research, so the selection of the nurse membership of the research team was easy. One of the nurses was a nursing faculty member at the local university, and there were two maternity nurses with a strong interest in community health and an eagerness to get involved. One way to diffuse my power in the project was to assign the recruitment of the CHW to the Dominican nurse research team as long as we agreed in principle how to do it. In consultation with the area public health director, they chose four of the most vulnerable and geographically representative neighborhoods in the city on which to focus the research. Ideally, we would have included rural areas, too, but it wasn't feasible for the amount of funding specified in the grant.

We walked the perimeter of each of these neighborhoods with the Dominican nurses, and while I was back in the United States, the Dominican nurses walked all the streets in each neighborhood asking people, "Who are the community leaders in your neighborhood? When you have problems in your neighborhood, who do you go to?" From there, the nurses found ten leaders, two women from each neighborhood and two men who were willing to participate as community research team members. From this point on, they are called community health workers, or CHWs, although they did not have any prior training in health care.

The training of the nurse/CHW research team included some didactic context and historical background of our research. We named the steps in the process of research in general, followed by the steps and process in our community-based participatory research project. We discussed ethics in research and the informed-consent process. Then we discussed the details of administration: payment, schedules, work expectations, and dates and times for activities. One good power-leveling decision was to design a subcontract budget from the Dominicans, because it meant the Dominicans had their own budget to manage. This was more complex (and time consuming!), but it was much more empowering for the Dominicans. Of course, we all had to stay within the budget, but they had some decision-making power, which was a great leveler in terms of shared decision making.

One of my early mistakes during the training phase was about study personnel. Both my own prior experience with CBPR, as well as the advice of an expert nurse researcher consultant on the grant, caused our over-recruitment of CHWs for the research team because of expected attrition. We assumed some CHWs would not show up or some would decide to drop out during the training session. In fact, this did not occur. So we had more CHWs than we needed or could afford. This was very difficult emotionally because of the Dominican cultural emphasis on positive social relations, and we had to essentially let go half of those we had recruited. To address this, on the last day of the training, we had a goodbye party for the CHWs who would not be continuing on the project. The Dominican nurses suggested we name them "understudies," maintaining their contact information in case of need later in the project. (Later on, we did need to use an understudy, because one of the CHWs did not perform well, and we had to make the difficult, but correct, decision to let her go.) We invited the understudies on the following trip when we presented their research ethics training certificates to all of them, about which everyone was very proud (see the section on research ethics training).

In the original plan for the study, training (Aim 1) came first, followed by the conduct of focus groups and interviews (Aim 2). But I discovered that the didactic part of the training needed to be followed right away by the application part for it to be effective. Given the fact I could only come to the site for 1 or 2 weeks every few months, we did some training, and then conducted the focus groups each visit. This method is really counter to the accepted practice of analyzing the data while you collect it, and I knew this might be a serious criticism of the research. I made a decision that it was more important to uphold the principles of CBPR, and that the team should analyze the data together. Therefore we collected the data at each of my visits until it was completely collected. Only then did we hold a whole separate training visit for analysis, to be discussed in more detail in the analysis section.

In the scientific literature about focus groups, there is a good argument for creating homogeneity of the groups (Morgan, 1997). In our study, we designed homogeneity of focus groups by sex and age. We decided on three different categories of focus groups—men, women, and adolescent girls— and we would conduct these in each of the four neighborhoods, resulting in 12 focus groups. We anticipated that because complications and death in mothers and babies carries great intimacy and emotional weight, it made sense that some women might tell stories with a rich and deeper background in private than they would have the time or willingness to tell in a focus group. That is why we decided to choose a participant from each group who might want to be interviewed individually after the focus group. This was the rationale for 12 individual interviews.

We also planned to ask any of the women in the focus groups who were pregnant if they would be willing to be accompanied to their prenatal visits and to be followed prospectively. This was the plan for participant observation. The research observer role was a role that the CHWs enjoyed and did beautifully. They documented the time of visits, the amount of time seen, and the situation of each person. We did not ask them to enter the room with the physician, both because of confidentiality, but also because we wanted the observations to be anonymous. Waiting rooms are public spaces, but observing the physician–woman encounter, without the knowledge or consent of the physician, would have been unethical. Also, if the physician agreed, we were sure that the activities of the visit would have been different than if an observer were not there. The observations were useful to affirm what we were hearing in the focus groups. This triangulation of qualitative methods verified the information we were getting from self-reported data.

RESEARCH ETHICS TRAINING AND
INSTITUTIONAL RESEARCH BOARD APPROVAL

At the commencement of the study, the first priority of the training was research ethics certification. Before the CHWs were even recruited, we worked with the nurses to become certified in research ethics. After the CHWs came on board, we spent the entire day at an Internet café, and each of the CHWs received the training in research ethics from Family Health International (FHI) 360, in Spanish (Rivera, Borasky, Rice, & Carayon, 2009). Half the group of CHWs came in the morning, and half the group came in the afternoon. None of the CHWs had ever used a computer before. It was a challenging day, but one of which we all felt proud; we stayed until all had successfully passed their certification test. I thought we would need to handhold the CHWs through the intricacies of the Belmont report, but it was not so. The idea of ethics and justice in research was readily understood. There were just more issues with navigating a mouse and a computer for the first time.

I sent the evaluations to FHI 360, and they issued certificates of completion that I presented to each CHW on the following trip. This worked really well, and FHI 360 has French, Portuguese, and English versions for community researchers to get certified in research ethics (Rivera et al., 2009). It is part of FHI 360's capacity-building service, located on the "services" menu on their website (www.fhi360.org).

Of course, prior to starting the project, institutional review board (IRB) approval from the university was required. Our application had a number of complex components to it. First, there had to be English and Spanish versions of every consent form. A letter from a Spanish speaker uninvolved in the research needed to affirm that the Spanish was an accurate translation, as required. Also, because our study participants included adolescents, there needed to be consents from their parents/guardians as well as the adolescents themselves in English and Spanish. There was also a separate consent for the men.

The most challenging part of the IRB application was that, for federally funded projects, you must have IRB approval, not only from the university where you come from, but also at the site where you will conduct the research. For hospitals used to research, this is time consuming, but procedures are well established. The hospital where we were located was not a research hospital and had never had research conducted there, let alone international research funded by the U.S. National Institutes of Health (NIH).

Sometimes I felt overwhelmed by all these regulations, but in practice, the officer at NIH referred me to a person who knew how to do this, and he explained it quite simply and directly with all the requirements. There is a form from the Department of Health and Human Services (DHHS) that is an IRB/independent ethics committee (IEC) registration. It includes the name of the chairperson and a roster of the IRB members, including their specialty and affiliation. The ethics committee must also include members who are not scientists. There are rules about conducting meetings, maintaining minutes, and so on. The officer explained it to me, so we organized this and created a hospital ethics committee in the Dominican Republic for this proposal with the medical director and the hospital chief administrator, with the idea there might be other proposals in the future. Once we had done this and documented it, we received federal-wide assurance right away (Office of Health and Human Services, 2014). It was very straightforward, but it took time. I suspect the biggest challenge at the site will be the ongoing meetings and maintaining minutes into the future.

Another lesson we learned early was related to the grant reviewers' concern with our human subjects protections plan. Reviewers required I make a plan to put in place in case any of the interviews were so psychologically traumatic for the participants that professional help would be in their best interest. Conferring with my Dominican professor colleague, we enlisted the services of a Dominican psychiatrist who would see any participant gratis in case she or he needed counseling after reliving a traumatic experience by means of our interviews. We did actually refer one of the participants who had lost her mother in childbirth when she was a little girl, but she turned down the offer to see the psychiatrist.

Another required regulation was a letter from someone who was not part of the study and who didn't work for the hospital. The IRB staff explained that they were interested in verifying whether the viability for the implementation, application and development of the project in the selected population was sufficiently high and reliable. Essentially, the IRB wanted a person from the local environs to affirm the feasibility of the project. Fortunately, I knew a Dominican colleague in the United States who had been a provincial coordinator of health programs in the same province we were working in, and he kindly read the proposal, agreed it was feasible, and wrote the letter. None of this was insurmountable, but just as with forming an IRB in another country, it took several months after we received the grant to get underway. At the time, all these procedures seemed enormous and overwhelming, but I learned a tremendous amount just by doing it. I felt like a pioneer, but I also always felt cautious, waiting for the "other shoe to drop," hoping that I did everything correctly.

RESEARCH TEAM TRAINING

The training included didactic content on focus groups and interviews. I had an excellent manual in Spanish published with United States Agency for International Development (USAID) support (Debus, 1995). The team observed a simulated focus group and semistructured individual interview. Then they practiced using a moderator interview guide to conduct a focus group, followed by an individual interview guide. The nurses were much more confident than the CHWs and were the ones who practiced interviewing and focus group guides. I had this idealistic notion that everyone would be a moderator, but the CHWs were intimidated by this idea and did not want to take on the moderating role.

It turned out that it was better for the nurses *not* to moderate the groups and interviews because some participants knew them as nurses, and we could observe by eye contact that participants were cautious about responding to the question about the care they had received in the maternity ward. After the first focus group, we had the usual worry: Are people telling us what they think we want to hear? As a group, we decided the U.S. researchers would moderate the focus groups and interviews from then on. It was another example of in-the-field decision making, based on the reality of what was happening before us. As usual, I hoped I was making the right decision; in this case I was.

We had created recruitment protocols, and we "practiced" doing recruitment. We planned for the actual recruitment of the research participants of the first neighborhood with dates on printed "invitations" for the conduct of the focus groups for women, men, and adolescents. During the actual recruitment, we tracked those not at home as well as those who did not wish to participate. On the advice of a statistician friend, we took notes about the homes of those who were not home or did not want to participate to get an idea if there were visible differences in the economic status of the nonparticipants (e.g., Were their houses made of wood or cement?). Because a randomized sample was not feasible, we wanted to be able to document if there were any reason that the nonparticipants were more likely to be better off economically. This would give us a sense of whether our samples were skewed by economic differences. They were not.

DATA COLLECTION

At the CHWs' suggestion, we formed "brigaditas" (brigades) of researchers, nurses, and CHWs in each of the three groups. It worked beautifully. We met together at a central point in the first neighborhood, and we fanned out in three different directions to begin recruitment per every third house. For the male sample, the male CHW used a snowball technique because we wanted to specifically find men who had experienced perinatal loss of the mother or newborn. In our recruitment process initially, we did not find enough males who had experienced loss of a close female relative (spouse, sister, mother, etc.) during childbirth. Alas, however, there were ample numbers of men who had experienced newborn loss. Therefore, we decided to expand our eligibility criteria to include men who had experienced newborn loss as well as maternal loss. Then we had no trouble at all finding eligible and willing male participants.

For the participant observation arm of the study, we also recruited pregnant women for the prospective sample. Of necessity, this became a convenience sample because not enough women in the focus group samples were currently pregnant. We recruited some women in the designated neighborhoods who were pregnant who agreed to be observed, and the CHWs took notes using a form we created to make sure they consistently observed the same things at each visit.

The Dominicans selected the sites for the focus groups. The first one was in a community center that was small, hot, and *noisy*. We lost some audible data because of ambient noise; the site was a mistake. We treated this as a learning experience for selection of sites for the future neighborhoods, and we never had that problem in the other sites.

For the transcription of the audiotapes, we hired a Dominican nurse not involved in the study nor on the maternity ward, who transcribed all the data in Spanish. One benefit was the lower cost than a U.S.-based transcription service. Another benefit was that the transcriber knew about health care, knew the culture, and could understand the Dominican local way of speaking, which tends to be fast, stream-of-consciousness, and informal, with a lot of slang.

DATA ANALYSIS

Data were collected between August 2008 and March 2009. The analysis phase began in March 2009 and was completed in January 2010. In March 2009, I traveled to the Dominican Republic specifically to do training with the team in qualitative analysis. The process was daunting—a team with vastly different educational preparation, two languages, and no previous qualitative research experience or research experience at all, with the exception of myself. We began by reading, coding, and creating a code list with definitions. We did all the analysis without qualitative data management software because none of the CHWs had personal computers or knew how to use one and it would have added another layer of expense and complexity to an already complex process.

One of the field notes captures the initial meetings for analysis:

> Initially D. and S. had many things to say and concerns about the codes. It was initially very chaotic with both wanting to speak over the others. ... The CHWs stated that they were in agreement with all of these decisions, but rarely spoke. B. was able to follow the discussion the most, K. and N. the least. What stands out the most for me, is that their ability for analysis is becoming more complex. In general they think concretely, for example, they have difficulty extrapolating a generality or summary statement of the examples. But they also understand when the examples don't fit the terms they have, and are passionate about having it right. ... The group worked fantastically, with insight and creativity for about 2 hours. Then all began to crash. They had a harder time seeing another's point of view, understanding concepts and becoming more and more attached to their particular opinion. We took a break. But the last hour the nurses used their authority and power more and more as evidenced by louder and louder voices, discussing more and more technical/medical types of points and overriding the community members. In the end we had to agree to disagree on certain phrases and some were only set to rest when E. said, "This is the way it should be"—culturally very interesting.

Based on these very real challenges before us in analysis, I made a decision to separate our analysis team into two groups, the nurses and the CHWs. Each group was asked to discuss the codes and begin to look for ideas and themes in their data across all the focus groups and interviews, neighborhood by neighborhood. At the end of each afternoon, the groups would come together and share what they discovered, and we taped the discussion about the shared understanding. This in turn was transcribed in Spanish. At this point, we were at the step of summarizing the content and identifying the central ideas. According to Sandelowski and Barroso (2003), our findings at this point were midway between closest to the data and farthest from the data.

By the visit in August 2009, we began the process of local dissemination first, to return to the neighborhoods and verify that what we had been hearing was valid and not some strange aberration of a particular sample. Each of the CHWs from each neighborhood and one of the nurses put together the presentation for the neighborhoods. This was also a step to ensure rigor, to have each of the neighborhoods hear the summaries of the focus groups as a way of member checking. Also, from an ethical point of view, it was very important for us to present our preliminary findings first to the people affected. So much research is collected and then never shared among the people affected. The practice maintains the status quo when knowledge is generated and then not shared.

These four neighborhood meetings were very well attended, ranging from 26 to 76 attendees. My sense was that each CHW should present the findings to his or her community. This was an example where I, as PI, should not be the person to present the findings; on this we all quickly agreed.

A particularly illustrative example of the CHWs' presentation happened in front of a big group of community members, consisting of 76 people. The persons invited to the meeting included all the participants in the focus groups and interviews as well as heads of local organizations, church groups, the mayor, the director of the primary health care clinic, and others who were interested. The CHW really wanted to do a PowerPoint presentation of the findings from her neighborhood. She had never done a PowerPoint presentation before, but she felt it was very professional and wanted to try it. One of the student research assistants from my university helped the CHW put together the graphics for her presentation.

We arrived at the outdoor community area of a public school to set up for the presentation. It was hot, mid-afternoon. We were busy hanging a sheet over a rope line to serve as a makeshift screen to show the presentation. Shortly after turning on the computer, the electricity went off in that section of the city. Frantic that she would not be able to give her presentation using PowerPoint, the CHW implored several friends in her community to fetch a generator. Seventy-six people were waiting in the open air, while two men on motorcycles went off to locate a generator. About 10 minutes later, they returned with one, and they started it up. The noise was deafening, much like a gas-propelled lawn mower. It was clear this was not suitable to give a presentation as no one could hear anything. The CHW, with encouragement from the team, made the presentation directly to the audience, just speaking without any technological support. She did an excellent job, and she was terrifically proud. I daresay it was better than a PowerPoint presentation would have been, because rather than being distracted by the slides, she spoke from her heart about what she knew.

Although there were individual differences by neighborhood, all four community meetings presented essentially the same messages, and these are reported elsewhere (Foster et al., 2010a). After each of these neighborhood presentations, which were conducted by the CHWs and nurses, the audience was questioned, "Does this presentation represent your experience?"

The responses by the audiences in all four neighborhoods were overwhelmingly affirmative. In fact, neighborhood residents stood up with urgency, wanting to tell their own personal stories, confirming the distrust toward health personnel regarding their perceived negligence. In one neighborhood alone, there were 50 suggestions from the audience for improved care in the hospital and 11 recommendations for the health system. While this volume of response was affirming that our findings did in fact illustrate the knowledge, attitudes, and beliefs in their neighborhoods, the volume of response was much more muted when we asked, "How can you participate with us to work for change in the hospital?" It was difficult to know if the question gave pause to the audiences because they had never considered they could be part of the solution or whether it was just easier to provide a litany of complaints about care they received than to volunteer to change the situation. Nevertheless, after all four meetings, there were 15 members from these communities who agreed to volunteer with the health providers from the hospital to improve care.

After these neighborhood meetings, the U.S. researchers met and proposed another layer of interpretation from the data, informed both by the global literature on maternal mortality and feminist critical theory. We shared this interpretation with the entire research team on another visit, and after input and edits from them, we prepared to present this study to the hospital personnel.

DISSEMINATION

The next priority was to disseminate our findings in the hospital that was the very location of numerous complaints. It was critical that the presentation have the correct tone and that it be about working together and not just about accusing the hospital of poor care. The research team came to realize how much we had listened to the community, so it would be important to create a presentation in which the hospital personnel could listen effectively to them. The Dominican team loved the idea of a skit or drama to present the findings. The presentation provoked fear and anxiety among the nurses and the CHWs, so we dedicated the better part of two visits in preparation and rehearsal for this presentation. The following excerpt is from the field notes:

They [the community volunteers] had good responses.... I realized how many skills are required for research...and good presentation style and performance are among them. So I did a fair amount of coaching, like walking to the back of the room to make sure community folks could be heard, making people slow down. But what a testament to the community's passion that M. narrated her story aloud, memorized, and not one word read or notes examined. My only job was to change slides. S. did a lot of the narration, but each team member had a vital speaking part, including a little drama about how mutual blame does not work, and working together being the way to solve the problems. M. and G. stood at either end of the raised platform and read aloud two of the most heart-wrenching stories, one from a male participant and one from a female. B. brought up the idea of cuña, (Dominican Spanish word for social connections that can bring privilege) and read two brief statements from the community about what cuña is. Then S. finished by saying if everyone treated people with equality and responsibility, there would be no need for cuña. She read aloud the WHO passage about working with individuals, families and communities. We ended with possible suggestions from the community about their roles, and then roles by the health providers. We opened it for questions.

The audience was clearly tense. They had sort of groaned when cuña was brought up. One of the nurses stood up and said she had been working in the ICU for 20 years, and that they took good care of patients and that they did not use cuña. She went on quite a bit, clearly angry and defensive. So one of the community volunteers stood up in reply. He said that he was no stranger to the health system, having served as a paramedic for 15 years. He mentioned that precisely it was this nurse when he had knocked at the door of ICU when his father was inside, and that this same nurse told him abusively to go away when he simply had a question about medicines he needed to purchase. Then the same nurse stood up again and gave this impassioned monologue about how much she cared for her patients and that tears fell down her face when they were sick. I said to her that I noted her passion, and that precisely we invited her to participate as a volunteer with us. She quickly said she was much too busy and could not volunteer.

F. on Labor and Delivery also stood up and said to the community that Cesareans were not just to be given out as the best care, that there was a need for medical indications. (One of the stories was that the women should have had a Cesarean but did not get one.) There were a few more comments, but in general it was clear that the audience felt uncomfortable, tense, and anxious. Then [Dr.] E. arrived, and he came to the front. He began a long, animated monologue, but he clearly used humor (telling stories of his early foibles as a young doctor not knowing how to do deliveries and the midwives and nurses helping him out). His back was to me and I could not keep up with the story, but it changed the whole tone of the meeting. People laughed. But he also made very specific, helpful points, about how the community could advocate for the hospital if they really understood the problems the hospital had with materials, with things budgeted for one thing and used for another. He invited the community volunteers to work with him and the Director of the Hospital, and to begin to look at the hospital's budget. He talks quickly and voluminously, so I did not catch all he said, but I remember, he used the exact phrase, that we had conducted, "un estudio fenómenal," [English: a phenomenal study— in the most positive sense of the word], and thanked us for the work.

Then, B.H. [hospital volunteer and Chair of the Hospital Ethics Committee] stood up. She has such poise, such grace. She spoke slowly and carefully about the need to work together. There was a period of quiet, a pause. Then K.M. stood up. She said she wanted to volunteer as part of the hospital to work with the community team, and she "exortó," [exhorted] others in the hospital to do the same. And then it was over, and J. gave another prayer, to close. As people left, somehow a paper had circulated, and we had 8 names and phone numbers of people from the hospital willing to volunteer.

From this meeting, we had a 15-person volunteer team of CHWs and nurses and physicians who became known as the Grupo de Salud [Health Group]. Over the course of a no-cost extension year, this group worked together and tracked 30 women during pregnancy, birth, and postpartum. This pilot was the action component of the CBPR. They worked together as a team using cell phones both for communication and for identity symbols: *We are all researchers working together.* I had not realized how powerful the use of cell phones would be in leveling the playing field. The outcomes of this research contributed to the selection of the hospital as one of the top ten hospitals chosen by USAID to become a Center for Excellence for Maternal Child Health, submission of Gates Foundation and NIH research proposals, nine U.S. national presentations, nine international presentations, and three peer-reviewed journal publications, with a fourth in press at the time of this writing. Neither proposal was funded, however.

Given the current climate of diminishing research funding, I continue activities within the partnership with student service learning and evaluation projects, and we continue to explore funding strategies using mobile phone technologies to improve patient–provider communication. The biggest challenge has been maintaining momentum of the team when there is a lapse between funded projects. The Dominican team is very willing to continue to work together with us, but without a budget for dedicated time, future research projects must simply wait.

SUMMARY

In many ways, the findings of the study did not differ from other research reports about the quality of maternity care in the Dominican Republic (Miller et al., 2003). The most significant result from this study was the successful application of CBPR to involve local community leaders and health personnel to engage and work together throughout the research process. They systematically inquired, documented, analyzed, and presented their findings to the communities affected, and this knowledge dissemination encouraged the mobilization of community members and health providers to form an ongoing working group to promote change for quality improvement.

Dedication to the research project produced very effective communication between research team members and built a team identity crucial to the success of CBPR. At the time of this writing, the partnership continues through U.S. university student service learning, but the sustainability of CBPR is still constrained by lack of research support. The conduct of this research project was an enormous learning curve for all involved, but it affirmed for me, once again, the value of the CBPR approach in generating new knowledge for positive change within communities who stand to benefit most.

REFERENCES

Debus, M. (1995). *Manual para excelencia en la investigación mediante grupos focales.* Washington, DC: Healthcom Academy for Educational Development.

Foster, J. (2004). Fatherhood and the meaning of children: Results of an ethnographic study among Puerto Rican partners of adolescent mothers. *Journal of Midwifery Women's Health, 49*(2), 118–125.

Foster, J., Burgos, R., Regueira, Y., & Sanchez, A. (2005). Midwifery curriculum for auxiliary maternity nurses: A case study in the Dominican Republic. *Journal of Midwifery Women's Health, 50*(4), e45–e49.

Foster, J., Burgos, R., Tejada, C., Caceres, R., Altamonte, A., Perez, L., & Hall, P. (2010a). A community-based participatory research approach to explore community perceptions of the quality of maternal-newborn health services in the Dominican Republic. *Midwifery, 26,* 504–511. doi:10.1016/j.midw.2010.06.001

Foster, J., Chiang, F., Burgos, R., Caceres, R., Tejada, C., Almonte, A., . . . Heath, A. (2012). Community-based participatory research and the challenges of qualitative analysis enacted by lay, nurse, and academic researchers. *Research in Nursing & Health, 35*(5), 550–559. doi:10.1002/nur.21494

Foster, J., Chiang, F., Hilliard, R., Hall, P., & Heath, A. (2010b). Team process in community-based participatory research on maternity care in the Dominican Republic. *Nursing Inquiry, 17*(4), 309–316.

Foster, J., & Heath, A. (2007). Midwifery and the development of nursing capacity in the Dominican Republic: Caring, clinical competence, and case management. *Journal of Midwifery Women's Health, 52*(5), 499–504.

Foster, J., Regueira, Y., & Heath, A. (2006). Decision making by auxiliary nurses to assess postpartum bleeding in a Dominican Republic maternity ward. *Journal of Obstetric, Gynecologic, and Neonatal Nurses, 35*(6), 728–734.

Israel, B., Schulz, A., Parker, E., Becker, A., Allen, A., III., & Guzman, R. (2008). Critical issues in developing and following CBPR principles. In M. Minkler & N. Wallerstein (Eds.), *Community-based participatory research for health* (pp. 47–66). San Francisco, CA: Jossey-Bass.

Miller, S., Cordero, M., Coleman, A. L., Figueroa, J., Brito-Anderson, S., Dabagh, R., . . . Nunez, M. (2003). Quality of care in institutionalized deliveries: The paradox of the Dominican Republic. *International Journal of Gynecology and Obstetrics, 82*(1), 89–103; discussion 87–88.

Morgan, D. L. (1997). *Focus groups as qualitative research.* Thousand Oaks, CA: Sage Publications.

Office of Health and Human Services. (2014). *Federal wide assurance.* Retrieved January 8, 2014 from http://www.hhs.gov/ohrp/assurances/assurances/file/index.html

Rivera, R., Borasky, D., Rice, R., & Carayon, F. (2009). *Research ethics training curriculum.* Research Triangle Park, NC: Family Health International.

Sachs, J. D. (2005). *The end of poverty: Economic possibilities for our time.* New York, NY: Penguin Press.

Sandelowski, M. (2000). Whatever happened to qualitative description? *Research in Nursing & Health, 23*(4), 334–340.

Sandelowski, M., & Barroso, J. (2003). Classifying the findings in qualitative studies. *Qualitative Health Research, 13*(7), 905–923.

Thaddeus, S., & Maine, D. (1994). Too far to walk: Maternal mortality in context. *Social Science & Medicine, 38*(8), 1091–1110.

Chapter Six

Participatory Action Research:
One Researcher's Reflection

Marie Truglio-Londrigan

*P*articipatory action research (PAR) is an approach and a process whereby the researcher listens to those who have lived the experience of the issue that is of interest. Therefore, this issue becomes a common interest that binds the researcher and the participants. The relationship building between the two leads to trust, engagement, and full participation where decision making and reflections are shared as the research is built, implemented, and evaluated. The purpose of this chapter is to present one example of a PAR, titled *Partnership for Healthy Living: An Action Research Project* with emphasis on one of the researcher's reflections. The chapter begins with an introduction on how the PAR project began and the reasons PAR was selected, a detailed description of the Partnership for Healthy Living Project in story format, and finally, reflections on the project as contemplated and presented by one of the researchers.

LAYING THE GROUNDWORK

Demographic data highlight the now commonly recognized fact that the world's population is aging. According to the World Health Organization (WHO, 2012), between 2000 and 2050, the proportion of the world's population 60 years of age and over will double from 11% to 22%, representing an increase from 605 million to over 2 billion. Moreover, this increase will be evident in low- and middle-income countries who will "experience the most rapid and dramatic demographic change" (WHO, 2012, para. 2). Many of these countries present morbidity and mortality data demonstrating evidence of infectious and parasitic diseases. Noncommunicable diseases, such as heart disease, cancer, and diabetes, along with the existence of multiple comorbidities, are in evidence in these same countries. A similar picture is observed in the United States. According to the Federal Interagency Forum on Aging-Related Statistics (2012), there were 40 million people aged 65 and over in the United States, accounting for 13% of the total population, in 2010; by 2030 this number is projected to be twice as large, growing to 72 million. As these older adults are living longer there is also a rise in chronic diseases such as heart disease, hypertension, stroke, asthma, cancer, diabetes, and arthritis. Along with these diagnosed illnesses comes the routine use of prescription and over-the-counter drugs (Federal Interagency Forum on Aging-Related Statistics, 2012). Despite living with multiple chronic illnesses and sustaining their health through the use of multiple medications, older adults in the United States do age in their communities. According to the Administration on Aging (AOA, 2012) report, 55.1% of the older non-institutionalized community dwelling population live with their spouses and 29.3% live alone.

Two researchers and nurse educators, Gallagher and Truglio-Londrigan (2004), both community health nurses with specialization in gerontology, saw this population aging trend in their practice and witnessed the confusion experienced by older adults and their families as they attempted to become aware of services in their communities and of how to access those available services. To address this issue Gallagher and Truglio-Londrigan (2004) engaged in a descriptive, exploratory study that incorporated focus group methodology. The purpose of this study was to gain a greater understanding of community-dwelling older adults' perceptions of community supports. Content analysis revealed two categories—knowledge and systems. Facilitators and barriers were identified for both of these categories. "Knowledge facilitators included life experiences and learning from one another. A major knowledge barrier was noted to be lack of awareness. A system facilitator was caring connections. System barriers included: complex connections, pseudo-connections, superficial connections, and cookie cutter connections" (p. 3). The outcome of this study offered qualitative evidence of the confusion many older adults, who are attempting to age in their communities, experience as they identify, access, and make available for themselves community support services. This confusion stems from a lack of awareness pertaining to what exactly is available for them, as well as a lack of understanding of how to access the community services. The results of this research generated more questions than answers for these two researchers. It was the result of this past research, however, that offered encouragement for these two researchers to continue in their quest for not only greater understanding about this issue but for ways to encourage and engage older adults in the development of strategies that would empower them in terms of gaining awareness, accessing, and making available for themselves community support services.

THE ROAD TOWARD PAR

Community-dwelling older adults have an awareness of the importance of informal social support offered to them by family and friends. They are able to describe multiple experiences where these family and friends are accessible and available to them for support in a wide variety of ways, including the offering of knowledge, time, and other forms of assistance that would help them in carrying out their activities of daily living, including instrumental activities. What was not as clear, for these same older adults, was their awareness of what formal supports in the community were available and how to access these community supports. These more formal supports are generally offered by local, state, or governmental organizations (public, private, and/or other local organizations; Lassey & Lassey, 2001). These formal support services supplement those provided by family and friends in instances where the family and/or friends do not have the ability, resources, expertise, knowledge, competencies, and/or skills (Krout, 1994). To address this area Gallagher, Truglio-Londrigan, and Levin (2009) developed, with the participation of community-dwelling older adults, a partnership that was driven by the application of a PAR design to make known what was unknown.

PARTICIPATORY ACTION RESEARCH

Whyte (1989) noted that the traditional way of conducting research is different from PAR and that "PAR is a type of applied social research that contrast[s] with what probably is the most common type, which I call the 'professional expert' model" (p. 368). In PAR, the researchers are aware that they are not the experts, and that, for research to unfold in a way that would address a practical reality-based issue, there must be a partnership with the people or the population of interest who has experienced the issue. This partnership is one of collaboration, trust, and sharing between the "researcher and researched: blurring the line between them until the researched becomes the researcher" (Baum, MacDougall, & Smith, 2006, p. 854). With PAR, those who are researched are active participants and they share in the decision making about the topics to be researched, data collection, and analysis. In essence, they are active in seeking change to improve practical issues (Baum et al., 2006). This idea of partnership and sharing is further described by Reason (1998, p. 1), who noted that this research is "*with* and *for* people rather than *on* people." According to Speziale and Carpenter (2007), one of the significant aspects of PAR is based in this collective partnership because it seeks to "empower those who are part of the process to act on their own behalf to solve real world problems" (p. 327). Furthermore, these same authors note that in PAR there is emphasis on a partnership that is reciprocal in nature as each works together toward sharing knowledge and information, thus empowering the other. This, for most researchers, may not be in their traditional worldview as they are not typically asked to come to the research endeavor on a level playing field. Researchers must let go of their "power" and listen and learn through "interactions between researchers and participants, and giving voice to those who would otherwise not be heard" (p. 330).

Gallagher and colleagues (2009) chose PAR because their major intent was to engage and partner with community-dwelling older adults knowing that this engagement would enable the researchers to:

- Engage with community-dwelling older adults to come to know and understand their perceptions of formal supports and the barriers that inhibited them from accessing and making use of services that may be available to them. As these older adults share their stories and perceptions, information, which was unknown to the researchers, becomes known as older adults share information that has the potential for action and change.
- Engage with these same community-dwelling older adults through every step of the development, implementation, and evaluation of the community-based programs (the interventions) and the PAR.

The PAR endeavor noted here offers the researchers another way to conduct their research. It is a method different than the traditional research approach. The essence of this particular PAR endeavor was to engage older adults so that they would be able to share their experience of living in the community where a need for community supports was left unmet. The PAR design offered insight into the lived experiences of older adults, which initially may not have been known to the researcher. Working with the older adults, in both the active development and implementation of the community-based program (intervention) and in the active development and implementation of the PAR endeavor, assisted the researchers in observing any change or outcome such as knowledge acquisition and empowerment of the older adult, as they became more aware of community support services and developed the skills to both access these services and avail these services for themselves. Box 1 offers the story of this Partnership for the Healthy Living Project.

Box 6.1 *Partnership for Healthy Living Project: A Case Story*

The Partnership for Healthy Living Project was born out of an earlier research endeavor that highlighted the experiences of older adults as they attempted to access and make available for their use the more formal community supports that were supplemental to the informal supports provided by family and friends. The Partnership for Healthy Living Project was developed to establish a partnership that would facilitate action leading to change. Collaboration, trust, and engagement of all participants were foundational for the success of this partnership. The project was envisioned to be PAR in design and to assist the researchers to understand what was unknown for them as the community-dwelling older adults shared their lived experiences and difficulties as they attempted to understand their own needs, find community support services to meet these needs, and then ultimately gain access and make use of these resources so that they would be able to age successfully in their communities. To ensure the effectiveness of this PAR project, the data collected were qualitative in nature via focus groups and individual interviews. These focus groups took place throughout the project, and at the completion of the project, the individual interviews took place. Throughout the entire PAR project, community dwelling older adults were active, participating and sharing in the decisions at all levels of the project.

The initial stage of the Partnership for Healthy Living Project involved three researchers discussing the potential development and implementation of the Partnership for Healthy Living project and the potential communities to partner with. It was during these preliminary sessions that the researchers identified a particular town outside a major city in the Northeast. The reason this town was selected was because of the demographics of the town in terms of the aging trends of the population and also because of the economic, social, and health needs of the aging population.

An initial meeting was set up with the town officials. The purpose of this initial meeting was introductory. Discussion centered on the community-dwelling older adults and the needs of this particular population with emphasis on the barriers to community support services. The researchers also explained the importance of the PAR approach to these town officials with emphasis on the importance of the partnership and engagement of the older

(continued)

Box 6.1 *(continued)*

adults as being action oriented leading to positive change. The town officials were very supportive and it did not hurt that the town mayor was a long-time resident who happened to be a nurse.

The town officials suggested that the best location for this Partnership for Health Living PAR project to take place was at a local senior citizen nutrition site. These same town officials set up an initial meeting that took place at the nutrition site.

The initial meeting at the senior citizen nutrition site took place with the three researchers, the town mayor, and the official of the nutrition site being present. The researchers reintroduced the Partnership for Healthy Living Project emphasizing the PAR approach in terms of the partnership, engagement of the older adults, and focus on action toward change. The nutrition site official was in agreement that the Partnership for Healthy Living Project and the PAR approach were beneficial and gave consent for the project to begin. It was also decided at that time that only two of the researchers would move forward with the actual implementation of the PAR project. The nutrition site served 350 older adults between 60 and 90 years of age. Most received lunch via the nutrition van while 40 to 60 attended the lunch onsite daily.

Two information sessions were held at the site for the older adults. The purpose of the information session was to again present the project and the rationale for the project. It was explained to these older adults that the project required active participation and engagement at all levels and that shared decision making was key. Older adults who were interested in participating as full, active, and engaged partners signed an informed consent (approval was obtained prior to this from the institutional review board). Eight older adults signed the informed consent and all were White females who were 60 years of age or older. Of the eight participants, two lived alone. Three saw their children monthly or not at all.

Focus groups were held throughout the project. Participants engaged in these focus groups to discuss their lived experiences of attempting to access and use community resources and the issues that they encountered. In addition to voicing these issues, the focus groups facilitated conversations about ways in which older adults, individually and collectively, may develop strategies to counter these issues.

Several interventions were singled out by these older adults as potential strategies.

- First and foremost, these older adults appreciated focus groups as a means to voice their concerns and develop strategies to deal with these issues in an ongoing way. Based on their identification of the beneficial nature of these focus groups, the participants suggested that these groups continue through the entire project.

(continued)

Box 6.1 *(continued)*

- Second, the participants of the focus groups noted that they were not aware of many things and that this lack of awareness disempowered them. Because of their self-identification of lack of knowledge and awareness, they asked for implementation of two strategies—educational programs and the presence of a nurse that they could visit and ask questions of.
  - The older adults suggested that educational programs could take place just prior or after lunch at the nutrition site. Examples of education programs included dealing with health insurance issues, medications, and safety.
  - Their request for having a nurse come in stemmed from the fact that many of the participants noted the difficulty they had in understanding their chronic illnesses and that the complexity of their care was beyond their comprehension. (Fifty percent of the participants indicated they had a diagnosis of osteoarthritis, hypertension, insomnia, sadness, anemia, and/or hearing loss. In fact, 50% of participants indicated that they were diagnosed with ten or more conditions and 50% took four or more medications.) These older adults stressed how the management of their care was often a mystery to them, especially because their care plans and medications changed often. Their concern was that because of the complexity of their care and the changes that took place, as well as the complexity of the health care system, they were at a loss in terms of their needs, and what, if any, community resources were available for them. The participants noted that they needed someone they can go to and ask questions and help them navigate the community. All eight participants noted that they had a health care provider but that either the health care providers were very difficult to "get a hold of to ask simple questions" or the health care provider did not have knowledge of community resources. To counter this reality-based issue the outcomes of the focus group centered on the establishment of a program entitled "The Nurse Is In."
- The third and final strategy that these older adults identified for implementation was community projects that they wanted to develop, initiate, and evaluate on their own. These projects included contacting pharmacies in the town to negotiate home deliveries and also negotiate with the town officials to reinstall park benches throughout the town. There had been park benches, but these had been removed as teens were using them to congregate and/or use as props for skate board tricks.

At each step, in this Partnership for Healthy Living project, the participation, engagement, and action for change was evident. For instance, the

(continued)

Box 6.1 *(continued)*

implementation of the community pharmacy project involved contacting the four pharmacies in the town for medication delivery. The older adults composed a letter that advocated for them and spoke of their needs. Once this letter was composed, other older adults at the nutrition site signed the letter. The older adults then went out into the community to speak to the owners of each of the four pharmacies and to deliver the letter and their message using their own voices. The older adults found that one of the pharmacies did, in fact, deliver medications for a $2.00 fee; however, the older adults were not aware of this and consequently decided to have this information published in the nutrition site newsletter. They stated that this was the best way to share information with the other older adults. Of the remaining three pharmacies, two declined to offer the service, and one was interested; however, this pharmacy was not able to enact any change for no employee of the pharmacy drove, and in fact many biked to work.

Final reflections on the Partnership for Healthy Living Project are set out within the text of this chapter. It is important to note, however, that this initiative was conducted over 2.5 years and was marked by attrition. The group immediately experienced a loss of one individual who never participated in the first focus group. As the years unfolded other participants were lost due to death, moving in with family either to receive assistance or, in one instance, moving in with a daughter to help the daughter give care to the daughter's husband who was ill, and a hospitalization resulting in the older adult being admitted to long-term care.

An exit interview was conducted with the nutrition site official who noted the positive nature of the program; however, she was concerned over the limited number of individuals who availed themselves to the program. She did not understand why this was so. An exit interview with the one remaining participant also revealed the positive nature of the program for this participant. This participant too expressed dismay over the lack of participation among other members of the nutrition site.

The above case story, illustrative of the Partnership for Health Living Project, was adapted by permission of RCN Publishing from Gallagher and colleagues (2009).

REFLECTIONS

Any lived experience is complex and presents to those who are living the experience with questions. This is true as one considers what community-dwelling older adults must do to become aware of, seek out, gain access to, and make available for themselves community-based support services.

This raises the question: How do older adults problem-solve these complex reality-based issues? At the same time, one may ask: How do nurses take on this same challenge and assist these older adults? Furthermore, how do older adults and nurses dig deep and search for solutions that may not be immediately visible? According to Schön (1983), "In order to convert a problematic situation to a problem, a practitioner must do a certain kind of work. He must make sense of an uncertain situation that initially makes no sense" (p. 40). This certain type of work involves a process known as reflection. This process includes an awareness of an uncomfortable feeling or thought. Once there is awareness, then there must be the courage to engage in a critical analysis of the situation, including questioning, that may ultimately lead to the development of a new perspective and/or a new plan of action for change (Atkins & Murphy, 1993).

In PAR the reflective process is important. Reason and Bradbury (2001) and Bradbury and Reason (2003) talked of PAR and the connection between action and reflection. This is further exemplified by Baum and colleagues (2006), who identified that one of the ways that PAR differs from other research approaches is the reflection that takes place. They further note that, at the very heart of the PAR process, is "self-reflective inquiry that researchers and participants undertake, so they can understand and improve upon the practices in which they participate and the situations in which they find themselves" (p. 854). In fact, the PAR process is cyclic in nature "where the overall purpose of action is achieved as the participants collect and analyze data, then determine what action should be followed. The resultant action is then further researched and an iterative reflective cycle perpetuates data collection, reflection, and action" (p. 854).

How those who are involved in the PAR process engage in actions toward change, all the while integrating reflection, is a challenge. Schön (1983) offers insight into this challenge as he speaks to the processes of reflection-in-action and reflection-on-action. Reflection-in-action takes place as individuals "think about what we are doing" (Schön, 1983, p. 54) while they are doing it both individually and collectively, and while they are thinking about what they are doing, they continue with the process of "... evolving their way of doing it" (p. 56). In the case of PAR, this thinking about what is being done is a process that all individuals are aware of, accept, and become responsible for. Reflection-on-action in reflective practice is a process that takes place as moments unfold after the fact as those individuals who are involved in the PAR project "[think] back on a project they have undertaken, a situation they have lived through, and they explore the understandings they have brought to their handling of the case" (p. 61). This reflection-on-practice also may take place individually and/or collectively.

Reflection-in-Action and Reflection-on-Action

To begin these reflections, this researcher and author of this chapter makes note that reflection-in-action and reflection-on-action were in evidence throughout this particular PAR project. As noted in the case story, focus groups were carried out throughout the entire project. These focus groups were critical for the building of trust between the researcher as a participant and the older adult as a participant. In addition, the focus groups were instrumental in building trust between and among the participants themselves. There was, however, another positive outcome for these focus groups. This outcome was in the reflective work that began to take place. In these focus groups, all participants, whether they were the researchers or the older adults, would reflect on the reality-based issues they wished to work on, which issues were the priority, what their plan of action would be, and how they would implement and evaluate the plan. What became very clear was that, as the PAR project unfolded, there was a reflective component taking place in the focus groups. It was during these groups that the participants would discuss what was actually happening in the community as they were implementing their plans, evaluate what was happening, and reflect on what adjustments needed to be made to the intervention strategies that had been developed to address the issues. In essence, the reflection on what was happening took on an evaluative component that facilitated the development of alternative plans and strategies to address the issues being worked on. For example, in the case story presented, one of the community projects was working toward the community pharmacies making home deliveries. This entire project took time to discuss, develop, implement, and to evaluate the plan. The project began with the shared decision, among the PAR participants, to write letters to the pharmacies that the older adults used to obtain their medications. However, it was after reflective conversation during a focus group that it was decided that collection of signatures would be more effective to the success of the project. And, as further reflection-in-action unfolded, the actual visiting of the pharmacies to deliver the signed letters and personally voice their concerns was yet another shared decision collectively developed and jointly implemented.

Finally, reflection-on-action was in evidence at the completion of the PAR project as the remaining member of the older adult participants received an individual exit interview where that person was given time to reflect on the project. This same opportunity was offered to the nutrition site official. It was during these individual exit interviews that both individuals were challenged for their observation that there were a limited number of older adults willing to participate in the PAR project. It was this identification by these two individuals that caused this researcher to also reflect on the project to come to a greater understanding of the workings of this PAR project and how to develop such a project in the future.

A Researchers Reflection: The Experience of Conducting PAR

A reflection on this PAR project takes this researcher to the beginning when the researchers began the dialogue and work toward building the relationships that are so crucial to PAR. As previously indicated, the particular town was selected because assessments revealed the demographics of an aging community and, as such, the potential for the reality-based issues that had been illustrated in previous research findings (Kelly, 2005). It was important for the researchers to introduce themselves to the community and to seek out the town's political officials. It was the decision of the researchers to first contact these political officials because they felt that these officials would have their fingers on the pulse of the community. The outcome of these initial meetings was very positive, as these individuals were the more formal leaders of the community who were able to offer insight into the town, the needs of the town, and the people of the town, and to guide the researchers in terms of where the population of interest resided, where they spent their day, what their needs are, and how best to access this group of community-dwelling older adults. This was of particular interest to the researchers who understood the importance of participant recruitment. They would have to recruit individuals who have lived the experience of seeking community support and would be able to share their experiences and, at the same time, experience a sense of ownership in the "proposed decisions" (Whyte, 1989, p. 368). Ultimately, it was the value of the sense of ownership that the researchers sought, not only as a means of enhancing continued participation by the older adults, but also to facilitate the process of learning, empowerment, and change among all participants (van der Velde, Williamson, & Ogilvie, 2010).

As the case story illustrates, it was these political officials who took the time to introduce the researchers to the senior citizen nutrition center and the official of the center. This formal introduction was important because it signaled to the nutrition site official that there had already been an acceptance of the researchers by the town officials and, thus, further facilitated the PAR process. This introduction also signaled gaining of entry into the program (Danley & Ellison, 1999; White, Suchowierska, & Campbell, 2004). The nutrition official met with the researchers and shared her intimate knowledge of the participants of the nutrition site and offered thoughts and suggestions as to the best way to access the population of older adults. Questions such as the following were asked: What is the best way for the researchers to be introduced? How can the researchers work with this particular group of older adults? What is the best means of communication? There were also logistical questions such as: What are the best days or times? What is the best location for privacy in the nutrition site? In essence, the political officials were informants who directed the researchers to the nutrition site official, who was the gate keeper who then led the researchers to the potential participants (White, Suchowierska, & Campbell, 2004).

The nutrition site official, as the gatekeeper, felt that the best way of gaining entry, access, and acceptance by the population of older adults was by a formal introduction at the site during lunch time and that she, an accepted and trusted member of the nutrition program, would introduce the researchers, who would then explain their presence. Again, this seemingly simple act of introduction held tremendous influence in the early stages of the partnership development between the researcher and the older adults as potential future participants (Danley & Ellison, 1999; White, Suchowierska, & Campbell, 2004). Reflections on these early steps informed this researcher that the time it took to make these contacts and to nurture them was foundational to the PAR process. For example, the approaches that the researchers used in this PAR project were systematic, leading to the outcome of gaining access and hopeful acceptance by the potential participants. The rationale for this approach was to slowly build a rapport and trust with all individuals that the researchers came in contact with, knowing that trust is a precondition of any partnership (Kang, 1997). When there is trust, there is more likely to be open communication (Butterfoss, 2007). Open communication tends to lead to greater sharing of information, engaging in self-disclosure, and sharing lived experiences. Trust, as a concept, is essential in the PAR process as the participants reveal information that may be sensitive (Dorr Goold, 2001).

The two researchers did attend the nutrition site program and were introduced by the nutrition site official. The researchers spoke to the entire group and gave a brief introduction in terms of who they were. The researchers also highlighted their previous research and presented to the potential participants their findings concerning how community-dwelling older adults frequently described difficulty in knowing what resources were in the community, how to access those community support services, and how to avail themselves of those services. The researchers stressed that a program, to be developed at their nutrition site, was not actually developed as of yet for a very good reason. The researchers further explained that any program development and implementation would be based on what they, the older adults who wished to participate, would tell the researchers. Thus, it was continually stressed that this was not an endeavor where the researchers would come in and decide what the issues were and what needed to be done and do it. Rather, it was to be a partnership between the researchers and the older adults, who would collectively decide on the best courses of action for the issues they identified. This exemplified the words of Kelly (2005) who stated "PAR changes the relationship between theory and practice by producing knowledge not only for its own sake but also to produce change" (p. 66). Essentially, it was explained that they were to "play more active roles than simply those of passive informants" (Whyte, 1989, p. 369). Being clear about this very important role to be played by the participant was important so that those individuals who displayed an interest clearly knew and understood the importance of the partnership and the type of collaboration that was necessary (Danley & Ellison, 1999). This introduction to the actual senior citizen participants was successful for there appeared to be buy-in, and there also appeared to be a real interest.

The case story presented here offers a glimpse of how the focus groups were formed. Those who did participate were very verbal and very action oriented. Reflections on the PAR project provide a story of knowledge attainment, empowerment, and change previously noted. The learning process that took place was not unidirectional but bidirectional between the participants and the researchers (Woodward & Hetley, 2007). Further reflection on the PAR project, however, revealed to this researcher that it was more than bidirectional—it was multidirectional, as learning and knowledge took place between and among all individual participants and researchers alike. In essence, the words of Danley and Ellison (1999) hold true when they stated, "If knowledge is power, then sharing knowledge is sharing power. For PAR to achieve its aims, sharing power among team members is essential" (p. 18).

A question this researcher poses is: Why was there such limited participation? The attrition of older adults in this project was glaringly evident; however, given the vulnerability of this population, this is understandable. Danley and Ellison (1999) carefully discussed the idea of fluctuation in participation and noted "A steady group of representatives is advocated... continuity should promote cohesion, the building of trust, sharing of power, and research outcomes. However, this is not always possible" (p. 5). This researcher has reflected on this many times and has come to the realization that there may be a wide variety of factors that hindered older adults from actively participating in our PAR project.

First and foremost, the two individuals who were interviewed at the end of the project noted that the use of the nutrition site may not have been the best venue. Their belief, upon reflection, was that the nutrition site might actually be viewed as a place to socialize and have fun and therefore may not have been seen as a place where health issues were discussed and addressed. It is a place to get away from and not face the starkness of some realities. This offers a glimpse as to what the ideas, values, and beliefs were of the nutrition site participants in terms of their purpose for attending the nutrition site as being different than the goals and purpose of the PAR project.

The second reason offered by the participants, who were interviewed at project's end, had to do with a perception that some older adults may hold. They expressed concern that some older adults may have been afraid to participate in programs that had to do with issues and/or health because others may have interpreted their participation as an indication of a weakness on their part. If they, as nutrition site participants, were considered weak, then they would be vulnerable to the actions of other older adults. In essence, in this nutrition site there were informal leaders who had informal political influences. After carrying out this 2½ year PAR project, it became clear that those older adults, who had greater resources in terms of their abilities to care for themselves physically and mentally, had greater status among the older adults at the nutrition site.

Finally, there was a third reason offered, which had to do with confidentiality. Focus groups were key in this PAR project and, as such, communication, openness, and self-disclosure in terms of personal lived experiences was the norm. However, an outcome of such open communication was also leaving oneself open and vulnerable. This highlighted, for this researcher, the importance of ethical knowing and, in this case, the importance of confidentiality. This is a challenge for researchers and brings to bear the importance of how one emphasizes confidentiality in PAR to all participants, as well as sheds light on the type of orientation and education that may need to be offered to participants who may never have been active participants in a research project (Danley & Ellison, 1999). Ultimately, what was evident in this PAR project was the role that cultural and political nuances play in whether or not any endeavor is successful. To this end any researcher engaged in a PAR project must be knowledgeable of formal and informal politics as well as have cultural awareness and understanding of the population and/or community (Baum, MacDougall, & Smith, 2006; Lindsey & McGuinness, 1998), again illustrating the importance of assessments at the start of any endeavor.

Similarly, the "Nurse Is In" portion of the project was another example of the difficulties that became known in PAR scenarios. In this particular PAR project, the older adult participants decided that a strategy they wanted to pursue was an arrangement by which a nurse would come to the nutrition site on fixed days and times to work with older adults, assisting them with individual issues. This is presented in the case story section of this chapter. What was difficult for the researchers was how to actually implement this strategy that older adults wished to carry out. In the end, the nurse researchers became the nurses who worked individually with older adults who came to "The Nurse Is In" programs. Reflection on this raised concerns for this researcher. The enactment of a PAR is difficult, as the researcher embarks on the project and, at the same time, supports the participants with mentoring, coaching, and possible education. The blurring of roles may be an issue and is difficult to address. In this particular project, the researcher added another dimension—the role of a nurse delivering care. This further compounded this blurring. The nurse researchers were very conscious of this and were transparent about their roles and responsibilities at each and every segment of the project and frequently discussed this concern.

Ultimately, because of the experience of conducting this PAR project, this researcher would recommend the following in the future development of any PAR project. First, during the very early stages of "thinking about" a PAR project, deciding what resources may be necessary and how the researcher may access and make available these resources are crucial. For example, time is a critical resource for any nurse researcher in an academic setting. The time it may take to conduct population and community assessments and make contacts and develop trusting relationships in the community deserves consideration. In addition to time, there is the question that concerns the availability of other professional resources. Reflecting upon this PAR project, this researcher may have been able to contact other organizations in town and/or professionals to see if there could be an expansion of the partnership, whereby nurses from these organizations could have entered into the nutrition site and assumed the role of the nurse in "The Nurse Is In" aspect of the project. In addition, many of the issues that manifested themselves were issues where other professionals, such as a social worker, may have been useful. This illustrates how in PAR there is a need to be very aware of the community itself and the types of organizations and professionals present in the community who may in fact strengthen and expand both the PAR project and partnership.

This sheds light on the importance of intra-/interdisciplinary approaches to PAR. The importance of this intra-/interprofessional team work is reflected in the Institute of Medicine (IOM) publication, *Crossing The Quality Chasm: A New Health System for the 21st Century* (Committee on Quality of Health Care in America, 2001, p. 2), where there is discussion pertaining to the need for a "sweeping redesign." The need for this redesign may be put into practice in PAR if warranted. However, it is also clear to this nursing educator and nurse researcher that those in the academic environment must be vigilant about integrating intra-/interprofessional team work competencies in the curriculum as noted in the documents *Health Professions Education: A Bridge to Quality* (Greiner & Knebel, 2003) and the Quality and Safety Education for Nurses (QSEN) project (Cronenwett et al., 2007). The Interprofessional Education Collaborative (IPEC) (2011) also identifies and defines Interprofessional Collaborative Practice Competency. It is clear that there has been an enhanced interest in the notion of teamwork and the outcomes noted as a result of the decisions of the team, more specifically, interdisciplinary teams and the outcomes of these collaborative endeavors to build a "safer and better patient-centered and community/population oriented U.S. health care system" (IPEC, 2011, p. 3). Again, these works illustrate the synergy of PAR with interdisciplinary work. Ultimately, the intra-/interdisciplinary approach that engages the people plus multiple service providers, all as partners in the research process, increases the participants' abilities to "identify, understand, and effectively address key issues" (Hills, Mullett, & Carroll, 2007, p. 126).

Because the two researchers who were engaged in the actual work of the PAR project were nurse educators, there may be a possibility to develop a PAR project in the future by partnering with other schools within their university setting. In so doing, the PAR project would be interdisciplinary, and all professionals would work collaboratively with older adults. The intra-/interdisciplinary endeavor would be comprehensive and the professional expertise illustrative of the different disciplines may possibly address the complex needs of community-dwelling older adults in a more collaborative effort.

In addition to what has been described in the preceding paragraph, this researcher acknowledges that there was a need for greater attention and diligence to the assessment of the nutrition site itself, just as there had been an assessment of the community. For instance, the resources offered by this nutrition site were limited and did not offer much more than meals and a place where older adults may come to eat and socialize. The absence of resources, such as technology, that would strengthen its structure and enhance its processes was conspicuous. For example, during "The Nurse Is In" one of the older adults came with a medical insurance question. It quickly became known to the nurse that the individual had medical insurance that the older adult did not know of and never accessed it. When the nurse called the insurance program for information on how to enroll the older adult, the nurse was informed that the only way to begin the enrollment was to go online to the insurance website, download the form, fill out the form, and either mail it, fax it, or send it back to the insurance company as an attachment. Unfortunately, the older adult did not have the ability to gain access to a computer; the nutrition site had a computer but no Internet access. As a result, the nurse left the nutrition site, drove to her office, accessed the form from the insurance website, downloaded the application, then drove back to the nutrition site, helped the older adult fill out the form, and ultimately mailed it back to the insurance company. What has been learned from this endeavor is that, before the start of any PAR project, the researchers must carry out an assessment of the community and the particular site in which the PAR will take place. This is important so that there may be an identification of what resources are available or not available. If certain resources are not available, such as professionals or technology, these are challenges that need to be addressed.

CONCLUSION

The International Conference on Primary Health Care meeting in Alma-Ata, Russia (1978) saw the adoption of the Declaration of Alma-Ata. In this document, the need for action was articulated as noted in the ten declarations. The seventh declaration speaks of primary health care (PHC) and notes that PHC:

> Requires and promotes maximum community and individual self-reliance and participation in the planning, organization, operation and control of primary health care, making fullest use of local, national and other available resources; and to this end develops through appropriate education the ability of communities to participate. (Article 7, number 5)

PAR, is an example of how professionals, in partnership with the people they serve, may facilitate, support, enhance, coach, sustain, and enact those steps that have the potential for the realization of PHC. It is no wonder that in recent years PAR, as a research methodology, has been heralded as a progressive, positive, and essential research strategy for community endeavors. More recently, the World Health Organization (WHO) published *The World Health Report 2008: Primary Health Care—Now More than Ever* (WHO, 2008). This document presents four major reforms: service delivery, universal coverage, leadership, and public policy. Service delivery reforms are the focus in patient-centered care or population-centered care that actually places the people at the center of care. What better way to position the people we serve than at the center of care? The center can be a place where active participation by the people in partnership with professionals may lead to knowledge attainment, empowerment, and change.

REFERENCES

Administration on Aging (AOA). (2012). *A profile of older Americans 2011: Living arrangements*. Retrieved from http://www.aoa.gov/Aging_Statistics/Profile/2011/6.aspx

Atkins, S., & Murphy, K. (1993). Reflection: A review of the literature. *Journal of Advanced Practice, 18*, 1188–1192.

Baum, F., MacDougall, C., & Smith, D. (2006). Participatory action research. *Journal of Epidemiology and Community Health, 60*(10), 854–857.

Bradbury, H., & Reason, P. (2003). Action research: An opportunity for revitalizing research purposes and practices. *Qualitative Social Work, 2*(2), 155–175.

Butterfoss, F. D. (2007). *Coalitions and partnerships in community health*. San Francisco, CA: Jossey-Bass.

Committee on Quality of Health Care in America. (2001). *Crossing the quality chasm: A new health system for the 21st century*. Washington, DC: National Academies Press.

Cronenwett, L., Sherwood, G., Barnsteiner, J., Disch, J., Johnson, J., Mitchell, P., . . . Warren, J. (2007). Quality and safety education for nurses. *Nursing Outlook, 55*(3), 122–131.

Danley, K., & Ellison, M. L. (1999). *A handbook for participatory action research*. Boston, MA: Boston University.

Dorr Goold, S. (2001). Trust and the ethics of health care institutions. *The Hastings Center Report, 31*(6), 26–93.

Federal Interagency Forum on Aging-Related Statistics. (2012). *Older Americans 2012: Key indicators of well-being*. Washington, DC: U.S. Government Printing Office.

Gallagher, L. P., & Truglio-Londrigan, M. (2004). Community support: Older adults' perceptions. *Clinical Nursing Research, 13*(1), 3–23.

Gallagher, L. P., Truglio-Londrigan, M., & Levin, R. (2009). Partnership for healthy living: An action research project. *Nurse Researcher, 16*(2), 7–29.

Greiner, A. C., & Knebel, E. (2003). *Health professions education: A bridge to quality*. Washington, DC: National Academies Press.

Hills, M., Mullett, J., & Carroll, S. (2007). Community-based participatory action research: Transforming multidisciplinary practice in primary health care. *American Journal of Public Health, 21*(2/3), 125–135.

International Conference on Primary Health Care. (1978). *Declaration of the Alma-Ata*. Retrieved from http://www.who.int/publications/almaata_declaration_en.pdf

IPEC (Interprofessional Education Collaborative Expert) Panel. (2011). *Core competencies for interprofessional collaborative practice: Report of an expert panel.* Washington, DC: Interprofessional Education Collaborative.

Kang, R. (1997). Building community capacity for health promotion: A challenge for public health nurses. In B. W. Spradley & J. A. Allender (Eds.), *Readings in community health nursing* (5th ed.). New York, NY: Lippincott Williams & Wilkins.

Kelly, P. (2005). Practical suggestions for community interventions using participatory action research. *Public Health Nursing, 22*(1), 65–73.

Krout, J. (Ed.). (1994). *Providing community-based services to the rural elderly.* Thousand Oaks, CA: Sage.

Lassey, W. R., & Lassey, M. L. (2001). *Quality of life for older people: An international perspective.* New Jersey, NJ: Prentice-Hall.

Lindsey, E., & McGuinness, L. (1998). Significant elements of community involvement in participatory action research: Evidence from a community project. *Journal of Advanced Nursing, 28*(5), 1106–1114.

Reason, P. (1998). Human inquiry in action: Developments in new paradigm research. In P. Reason (Ed.), *Introduction* (pp. 1–17). London, England: Sage.

Reason, P., & Bradbury, H. (2001). Introduction: Inquiry and participation in search of a world worthy of human aspiration. In P. Reason & H. Bradbury (Eds.), *The handbook of action research* (pp. 179–188). Thousand Oaks, CA: Sage.

Schön, D. (1983). *The reflective practitioner: How professionals think in action.* New York, NY: Basic Books.

Speziale, H. J. S., & Carpenter, D. R. (2007). *Qualitative research in nursing: Advancing the humanistic imperative* (4th ed.). New York, NY: Lippincott Williams & Wilkins.

Van der Velde, J., Williamson, D. L., & Ogilvie, L. D. (2010). Participatory action research: Practical strategies for actively engaging and maintaining participation in immigrant and refugee communities. *Qualitative Health Research, 19*(9), 1293–1302.

White, G. W., Suchowierska, M., & Campbell, M. (2004). Developing and systematically implementing participatory action research. *Archives of Physical Medicine and Rehabilitation, 85*(Suppl 2), S3–S12.

Whyte, W. F. (1989). *Advancing scientific knowledge through participatory action research.* Sociological Forum, 4(3), 367–385.

Woodward, W. R., & Hetley, R. S. (2007). Diffusion, decolonializing, and participatory action research. *Integrated Psychiatric Behavior, 41*(1), 97–105.

World Health Organization (WHO). (2008). *The World Health Report 2008: Primary Health Care—Now More than Ever.* Retrieved from http://www.who.int/whr/2008/en/

World Health Organization (WHO). (2012). *Aging and life course: Interesting facts about aging.* Retrieved from http://www.who.int/ageing/about/facts/en/index.html

CHAPTER SEVEN

COMMUNITY-BASED PARTICIPATORY RESEARCH: LESSONS FROM THE FIELD

Bonnie H. Bowie and Lauren Valk Lawson

*B*ringing together a diverse group of community partners to work toward a common research goal for the benefit of the community can be both daunting and rewarding for the researcher. Community-based participatory research (CBPR) is not simply conducting research within a community; it begins with collaboration with community members to identify what is of importance to them. CBPR requires researchers to be open to the capacity that individuals bring to the process as well as a willingness to share leadership (Community-Campus Partnerships for Health, 2011). Community partnerships in CBPR come from a variety of sources such as service providers, clinics or mental health treatment centers, religious entities, governmental agencies such as local public health or housing authorities, and the people living within the community. What is special about CBPR is that it is a process that empowers the community partners to gain control over their own situation. Therefore, a fundamental difference between CBPR and other types of research is that the research questions originate from the community itself rather than the researchers (Minkler & Hancock, 2003). To be successful, academic partners need to listen carefully to community members, sort through myriad community issues, participate in meetings where community members may be at odds with each other, and maintain academic rigor without appearing omnipotent—all while moving a diverse group of people with varying opinions toward a common goal. What follows is a description of our experience with a CBPR project in a neighborhood in north Seattle, including unanticipated barriers, successes, and mistakes. It is our hope that by sharing this account of our experience, others may benefit from the rewarding practice of CBPR.

DESCRIPTION OF THE STUDY

Several authors have noted that the best community–academic relationships start with a foundation rooted in a prior engagement, whether it is volunteer experience, board work or, as is often the case in the nursing discipline, a clinical rotation (D'Alonzo, 2010; Minkler & Hancock, 2003). During Fall Quarter 2008, as a part of their community nursing clinical experience, a group of nursing students from our College of Nursing (CON) were completing a community assessment of the Lake City neighborhood and discovered "God's Lil' Acre," an outreach ministry for the homeless run by the Seattle Mennonite Church (SMC). This encounter was the beginning of a successful ongoing partnership between one of the authors (LVL) and a succession of both undergraduate and graduate nursing students working with SMC to provide and enhance services to the homeless in the Lake City community. Over the next year, it became apparent to members of the SMC and CON that there was a gap in services for the medically fragile homeless. For example, a long-time member of the Lake City homeless community was hit by a car, which resulted in internal injuries and multiple fractures to his legs. After 2 weeks in the hospital, he was discharged to the streets with no supportive services. Members of the homeless community and local service providers were outraged. This was one of several events that demonstrated the gap in health services for individuals experiencing homelessness for this community.

To address the issue of hospital discharge of homeless individuals to the street, many cities in the United States have opened medical respites. Traditionally, the term respite (or recuperative) care refers to providing a break for a caregiver of a chronically ill family member. However, in this context, respite care means providing adults experiencing homelessness with recuperative or convalescent services in a safe place away from the dangers of the street (Ciambrone & Edgington, 2009). Overnight emergency shelters do not allow clients to remain on the premises during the day. Sick or injured adults experiencing homelessness, such as the man described earlier, need a place where they can rest and recuperate, receive nutritious food, get assistance with dressing changes, receive general nursing support, and have a safe place to store needed medications. As SMC and our CON continued to work with other community agencies to provide services to the Lake City homeless, we began to talk about addressing the gap in recuperative services for this vulnerable population. To address the issue, it was evident that we needed to garner community support prior to implementing any services to ensure relevancy and sustainability of the project. There was also a possibility that some members of the Lake City neighborhood may not welcome the expansion of services to the homeless, feeling an expansion may attract more homeless people. CBPR provided the framework in which to investigate the possibility of the creation of a medical respite in Lake City because the process would engage existing and potential partnerships, and could enhance sustainability.

Early in our partnership with the SMC, we drafted a memorandum of agreement (MOA) between our CON and the SMC. This route provided an opportunity to identify expectations for each partner and to learn about each other as organizations. One of the community ministers at the SMC, Melanie Neufeld, was actively involved in developing community partnerships for advocacy for the homeless and to bridge relationships with the neighborhood of Lake City. During the initial planning meeting in spring 2011, we identified the need to first form a community advisory board (CAB) to guide the vision, mission, and research process, and Pastor Neufeld agreed to chair this group.

Forming the CAB

Within community health nursing, "community" can refer to any group of persons with a shared identity such as living in a particular neighborhood, belonging to a specific ethnic group, or sharing a medical diagnosis like breast cancer (Pharris, 2012). For this research project, the term "community" refers to those people living and working in the Lake City neighborhood or who have a vested interest in the well-being of the Lake City homeless population. We felt it was important for the CAB to be comprised of community members who could bring knowledge and expertise to the decision-making process, be representative of important stakeholders in the neighborhood, and be willing to work toward solving the problem of recuperative services for the Lake City homeless population. Therefore, in the beginning, we simply invited representatives from any agency or entity that fell within these general guidelines. There are many good resources available for guiding the process of forming and maintaining a productive CAB. An article we found to be particularly useful and illuminating was the article of Newman and colleagues (2011) entitled "CABs in CBPR: A Synthesis of Best Processes." Newman and colleagues (2011) identify three processes of CABs: formation, operation, and maintenance. We describe here our experience with each of these processes.

Formation

During the formation process, it is helpful to identify the purpose, function, and roles of board members. If the CAB is to effectively support a participatory research model, members need to be partners rather than advisors to the researchers (Newman et al., 2011). During the first year of the Lake City Homeless Project, membership was constantly changing as new players came and went, and we found it difficult to form trusting relationships among the board members as a result of the inconsistency. It seemed as though we were continuously starting over in establishing our purpose and decision-making process. On the positive side, we were able to recruit new members through a snowball approach by asking at each CAB meeting, "What additional information is needed?" and "What members from the community are missing?" When a CAB attendee suggested an agency that was not at the table, we contacted that agency to request a representative attend the next meeting. It was also challenging for us to let go of our academic expertise and engage with community board members as equals in the process. When we did treat CAB members as true partners and listened to their input, the result nearly always enriched the research approach, as will be seen when the IRB process is described.

Eventually, a core group of constant members emerged, and this group agreed to address the issue of board membership changes by identifying a constant group that represented the diverse interests of the community. CAB members felt that if we were to evolve into an effective decision-making board, we needed to close membership, at least for a time, at some point. Early achievements of the CAB include creating a purpose and mission statement.

Operation

Newman and colleagues (2011, p. 5) state that, "A key element of effective group process is the fair and appropriate distribution of power and leadership; however, balancing power among diverse partners who represent multiple levels of social hierarchy is challenging." Identification of a community partner as the CAB chairperson with the skills to navigate communication among a diverse group of individuals with different backgrounds and education is paramount to the success of the CBPR process. The appointment of our community partner, Melanie Neufeld, as chairperson improved the operations of the CAB and allowed us to level our roles as academics and researchers. In this leadership capacity, Ms. Neufeld brought her knowledge of the Lake City neighborhood that assisted in the identification of additional CAB members. Her background in social work also helped us identify members of the homeless community to participate in the CAB and to address potential barriers to participation, such as transportation and communication styles. Though there has not always been consistent representation from the homeless community at the CAB meetings, the ability to incorporate all individuals into the meeting was an important skill. A consistent method for decision making as a CAB is something that we have continued to struggle with. Because the underlying philosophy of CBPR is to create a research process where all are heard, early in the process we tried to implement a "mutual invitation" communication model during meetings. In this model, the chairperson asks each member to either "share," "pass," or "pass for now," when an issue is being discussed where input is needed from each member. This method worked well, but was not reinforced at subsequent meetings and faded into disuse. On the other hand, we have not experienced a situation where one CAB member dominated discussions and so have not felt the need to reinstate the mutual invitation method. In addition, our facilitator does an excellent job of ensuring all are heard during meetings.

Early in the establishment of the CAB, we also took time at a meeting to discuss working agreements. In particular, we made a list of what we felt was important for our communication process. The group identified the following elements of communication as most important to the smooth functioning of the CAB: respect, honesty, honoring everyone's voice, active listening, safety, and speaking one's own truth. We also agreed that we would engage in advocacy- and capacity-building activities. An example of one capacity-building activity is the training that was held on CBPR for the CAB members.

During early discussions, it was apparent that the CAB needed more information regarding the community of people for whom we were designing services. A clearer picture about them and their health would better inform the CAB in its mission. As a result, we presented a potential research project that would complete a demographic study of the homeless community, including their prevalent medical problems, utilization of health care services, and whether they would use recuperative care.

Maintenance

Two years into the establishment of the CAB, we have yet to finalize a consistent board membership; however, we are getting closer. A site visit to a more mature recuperative care program in California with a business model–type board provided us with several ideas for how our own board might evolve.

Through this site visit we discovered that we may want to recruit board members who bring skill sets such as fund raising, grant writing, and legal expertise. We have also begun to explore the possibility of transitioning our CAB to a board of directors to manage a medical respite.

Newman and colleagues (2011) recommend a process evaluation to assess group dynamics such as shared leadership, open communication, mechanisms for resolving conflicts, and trust and cohesion. We have not yet performed a process evaluation because our CAB membership has yet to stabilize. We did revisit our mission statement when the CAB reconvened at the beginning of the 2012 to 2013 academic year. Process evaluation has been a challenge to implement because the current focus and energies of the CAB have been on getting a respite model implemented.

Conducting the Research

As the CAB discussed the problem of providing recuperative services to the Lake City homeless, we realized we needed more information about the population for whom we were designing services. What were their prevalent medical problems? Where did they normally seek medical care? If we were to develop recuperative services, would they use them? And, what model of recuperative services would best meet the needs of this population? After reviewing the literature and speaking to several experts, we decided to use the Vulnerability Index© (VI) questionnaire. The advantages of using this instrument included widespread use with homeless populations throughout the United States, and it was created to be administered by lay people. Additional advantages included access to a national database for comparison of results, no charge for using the questionnaire, and the freedom to add questions for our specific population. The biggest disadvantage of using the VI was there was no reliability or validity data available at that time. And we discovered later that we did not have access to the national raw database, only the aggregate numbers. This meant we could not use inferential statistical methods to test for differences between our data set and the national or regional data sets but could only use descriptive analytical techniques. Our inability to use more sophisticated analytical approaches has made the publication of the results more difficult, and at this writing, we are still looking for an appropriate journal to publish the initial results of the VI survey.

During this time, the CAB created a research committee, which was a subgroup of the CAB, to oversee the research. The research committee was comprised of ourselves, the chairperson, two graduate students, and three members of the homeless community in Lake City. For the data collection phase, we paired a graduate student or faculty member with a member of the homeless community. As part of our CBPR process, we included community members on the research committee and as part of a research team to ensure the relevancy and sensitivity of the project. We also believed their involvement would assist us in locating homeless people in the neighborhood and in administering the VI questionnaire. We hired and paid the homeless community members through a program called Vital Jobs Workers, which is a program through the SMC to provide job experience and references for future work. As the research group met to work out the details of the data collection process, we began to write our application to the university's institutional review board (IRB).

Overcoming the Traditional IRB Process

Overall, the IRB submission and approval process took 8 months, about 7 months longer than anticipated. The first response of the IRB committee was that they must have misunderstood—surely, we did not intend to have members of the homeless community actively participate in the administration of the questionnaires as there were sensitive questions about drug and alcohol use and communicable diseases such as HIV and tuberculosis. In addition, the IRB was worried about coercion of homeless community members by their peers and a lack of knowledge regarding confidentiality and human subjects' issues. The IRB stated that if we wanted to use homeless people to assist in the data gathering process, they would need to go through the National Institute of Health Human Subjects Training. All of these concerns were valid and needed to be addressed; however, as community-based researchers, we also felt that the IRB lacked an understanding of this type of research approach. We then composed a long letter to the IRB explaining why it was so important to include members from the homeless community and why requiring these community members to go through traditional Human Subjects Training was unreasonable. Here is an excerpt from that letter:

> While it is unusual to include members of a community in a research process, particularly when subjects are being asked to reveal sensitive information, it is the consensus of the Community Advisory Board that subjects will be more apt to participate in the survey if trusted members of the community are present, such as the Vital Jobs Workers referred to in the application. In addition, the overarching purpose of Community Based Participatory Research is to perform research with

the community, rather than on the community. The Vulnerability Index was developed by the Common Ground organization in New York with the intention of being administered by both peers and other types of volunteers. The Index has been administered in this manner, without incident, in several cities across the United States (see the Common Ground website for more information: *http://www.commonground.org/*). Interestingly, because Community Based Participatory Research is a "different animal," the University of Washington now has a separate IRB committee to review CBPR applications.

We want to assure the committee that we will be working closely with the Vital Jobs Workers during this process and providing training on confidentiality and skills to avoid coercion. We are also asking them to sign a confidentiality agreement modeled after the Common Ground confidentiality agreement form. If at any time we feel one of the Vital Jobs Workers is not adhering to the confidentiality agreement, s/he will be dismissed from the project. We have also made the decision to hire two people who are no longer homeless, but are in permanent housing and have proven themselves to be capable of serving in this role through prior work [with] the pastor at Seattle Mennonite Church.

At one point in this process, we informed the research team that the members of the homeless community may not be able to participate in the data collection process as first envisioned. In other words, these members of the team would most likely not be able to be directly involved in administering the VI questionnaire. One of these members became very angry and walked out of the meeting. We realized at that moment how invested these community members were in the research project and how important it was to them. We also suddenly realized that the research project no longer belonged to us, but had become a shared process with our community members. We also realized that to maintain the trust and involvement of all of our community members, we needed to investigate alternative methods for Human Subjects Training that would meet the requirements of the university's IRB but were not aimed at a research audience. During this search, a resource that we found to be invaluable was a website from Community Campus Partnerships for Health (2011; www.ccph.info), which included several useful documents, including approaches to IRBs.

Through the assistance of Dr. Bonnie Duran at the School of Public Health at the University of Washington, we were able to connect with Dr. Eugenia Eng from the Gillings School of Global Public Health at the University of North Carolina (UNC). Dr. Eng graciously shared a Human Subjects Training module she and her colleagues had developed for nonacademic community-based research members. In a compromise reached with the IRB, we agreed to administer the UNC Community Member Human Subjects Training module with our research team members using an outside consultant to facilitate this process. In addition, we agreed that all subjects would be approached first by the graduate student or faculty to obtain verbal consent for the presence of the homeless community member during the administration of the VI questionnaire.

After receiving IRB approval, we scheduled a half-day meeting for the research team to participate in the training module. We felt it was important for the team to do the training together to enhance teamwork. This decision turned out to be important as we were able to talk through various scenarios that might present to team members as they were in the field collecting data. For example, what should the data collectors do if a subject appeared to be under the influence of drugs or alcohol? There were also several rich discussions about what it means to protect human subjects and confidentiality. The homeless members of the team were particularly enthusiastic participants, and their ownership of the research project was evident.

Data Collection and Analysis

After overcoming so many barriers with the IRB, we were pleasantly surprised when data collection went quite smoothly. By including homeless community members on the research team, we were able to locate several hard-to-reach homeless persons who agreed to answer the VI questions. For their time, participants received $10 worth of bus coupons. We were also able to recruit participants through flyers in the local homeless shelter and through word of mouth. The bus coupons were very popular with subjects and turned out to be an effective recruitment tool. The final number was 47, with 46 completed questionnaires.

Storage of the completed VI questionnaires in a secure place initially posed a problem. We did not want the graduate students transporting the questionnaires in their cars, nor did we want them left in a place that was not secure. In the end, we decided to store the completed questionnaires in the pastor's locked office in a locked file cabinet until they could be picked up and stored at the university. In this way, we ensured that the pastor would always be available as the work supervisor for the homeless members of the research team and data would not be collected after church office hours.

As the research team was reviewing preliminary results of the VI questionnaire, one of the academicians spoke to the group in technical, data analysis terms. One of the research team members, who was homeless, became very frustrated and angry when she was unable to understand what was being presented. We were reminded that we were now a part of a broader team of people with varying backgrounds and expertise. We apologized and adjusted our presentation accordingly.

Some of the most useful and significant information from the VI questionnaire was the demographic and medical problem descriptions of the Lake City homeless population, which enabled us to create a profile for the Lake City homeless. For example, a larger percent of our population were veterans (25.5%) as compared to the national average (18.4%), indicating a possible need to seek a more formal partnership with Veterans' Administration services. We also found that a majority of the study group was male (72%) and White (52%) and ranged in age from 28 to 66 years with an average age of 48.6 years. The average reported length of time homeless was 4.7 years with a range of less than 1 year to 19 years. The participants were more likely to experience substance abuse than the national average (78.7% versus 57.4%), and they were more likely to have conditions that put them at risk than the national average (59.6% versus 43.9%). (At-risk qualifiers included HIV/AIDS, cold weather injury, kidney or liver disease, visits to the emergency department 3 times or more in 3 months, age 60 or older, and/or a hospital patient 3 times or more in 1 year.)

Disseminating the Results

The first audience with whom we wanted to share the VI questionnaire results was the CAB. With the input of the research team, we prepared a PowerPoint presentation for one of our CAB meetings and also invited other interested members from the Lake City community. We were careful to assign roles to all members of the research team for the presentation, and we talked them through how the presentation would be orchestrated as a team. As an example, the PowerPoint slides contained fewer graphics, and statistics were explained simply. While most attendees found the information to be interesting and helpful, the presentation also stimulated more questions. Many attendees suggested other information that should have been or could be obtained from the participants, not realizing that we were bound by the constraints of what was contained in the IRB proposal.

Following the presentation to the CAB, the research team met again to talk about how to present and validate the information with members of the Lake City homeless community. Since most of these people visit the drop-in shelter regularly, it was decided to print out the PowerPoint slides and post them on the walls of the shelter. We also invited people to write comments on the slides. We were pleasantly surprised at the level of engagement in this process. Many people wrote comments, affirming our findings such as, "This is true about me" and "I wish there was a respite around here."

CONCLUSIONS AND LESSONS LEARNED

While using CBPR for creating recuperative services for a homeless community has been a gratifying process, it has also posed several challenges. Defining and clarifying roles has been one of the most difficult pieces of this process. As principal investigators we were used to being in charge of all aspects of the research process. Researchers are accountable to the research subjects, funders, and IRB and must take that accountability seriously. We found it difficult at times to let go of the need to be in charge and allow others to provide input into the research process. We admit that we did not achieve a completely egalitarian decision-making process during CAB meetings. There were times when we had to speak up in order to be in compliance with IRB or other regulations or constraints. However, having someone else facilitate the CAB meetings did allow us to be in more of a participatory role rather than a leadership role.

We think that one of the key elements to our success thus far was finding a community partner in the SMC with a similar philosophy and approach to working with vulnerable populations. As we studied each other's history, belief systems, and mission statements for the formation of the MOA, we discovered our many similarities. This process also provided us with a deeper respect for each other's organizations and work in the community. The MOA, along with our prior community partnership, were key ingredients in the formation of a trusting working relationship between the two main partners.

If possible, we recommend obtaining funding with flexible timelines built in. The funding for this project came from a private family foundation, and thus, we were able to adjust timelines and line items as needed. The process of CBPR is unpredictable and may or may not adhere to projected timelines. If applying for funding through a more rigid funder, such as a federal agency, build in as much flexibility as possible into the projected timeline.

We are writing this chapter as though we, the academicians and researchers, are of one mind set, and of course that isn't true. As researchers, we came into this project with different expertise, expectations, weaknesses, and strengths. Part of our journey has been learning to leverage our knowledge and strengths toward a common goal and learning to trust and appreciate the strengths each of us brings to the project, just as we have with our community partners. We have accomplished this task while trying to establish relationships with a variety of community agencies and members. We want to emphasize that it was not a completely seamless process; however, it has been a worthwhile endeavor. Sometimes, faculty take positions in universities where it may seem there is not a logical collaborator for one's research interests. In these instances, faculty may end up collaborating with seemingly unlikely colleagues. Our experience should serve as an example of unlikely, but potentially positive, collaborations. When we embarked upon this CBPR project, Dr. Bonnie Bowie had never done this type of research; most of her research experience had been in quantitative prevention science. Dr. Lauren Valk Lawson had extensive experience in public health nursing and had created a number of the partnerships in Lake City to provide students with a rich community health clinical experience. Dr. Bowie brought research skills, including grant management, research design, and data analysis. She also had an extensive background in health care administration and outcome measurement. Dr. Lawson was working on her DNP degree during the first 2 years of the project. She was able to use the community assessment piece of the project for her capstone course and drew on the CBPR expertise of faculty at the University of Washington. We want to emphasize that successful CBPR requires a variety of skills for successful implementation.

And finally, as stated previously, CBPR is not a quick process, but must be allowed to unfold over time with input from community members. Relationships with members of the community can be fragile, each person bringing his or her own cultural beliefs and experiences to the decision-making process. Time after time we were reminded that it simply doesn't work to rush this process. At this writing, we are 2 years into this research project and are just now finalizing the membership of the CAB and procedures to conduct business. When we started, we estimated it would take about a year to perform a community assessment prior to implementing recuperative care services for the homeless in this neighborhood, and we are just now in the final process of the service design. We estimate that it will be another 2 years before we have fully implemented and evaluated the planned recuperative care services. And we fully expect our plans to change and evolve over the next 2 years as the community we work with changes.

REFERENCES

Ciambrone, S., & Edgington, S. (2009). *Medical respite services for homeless people: Practical planning*. Nashville Respite Care Providers Network. National Health Care for the Homeless Council, Inc. Retrieved from http://www.nhchc.org/Respite/FINALRespiteMonograph.pdf

Community Campus Partnerships for Health. (2011). *Community-based participatory research*. Retrieved from http://depts.washington.edu/ccph/commbas.html

D'Alonzo, K. T. (2010). Getting started in CBPR: Lessons in building community partnerships for new researchers. *Nursing Inquiry, 17*(4), 282–288.

Minkler, M., & Hancock, T. (2003). Community driven asset identification and issue selection. In M. Minkler & N. Wallerstein (Eds.), *Community-based participatory research for health* (pp. 135–154). San Francisco, CA: Jossey-Bass.

Newman, S. D., Andrews, J. O., Magwood, G. S., Jenkins, C., Cox, M. J., & Williamson, D. C. (2011). Community advisory boards in community-based participatory research: A synthesis of best processes. *Preventing Chronic Disease, Public Health Research, Practice and Policy, 8*(3), 1–12.

Pharris, M. D. (2012). CBCAR: Methology unfolding. In C. P. Pavlish & M. D. Pharris (Eds.), *Community-based collaborative action research: A nursing approach* (pp. 1–30). Sudbury, MA: Jones and Bartlett Learning.

CHAPTER EIGHT

A University–Tribal Community-Based Participatory Research Partnership: Determining Community Priorities for the Health of Youth

Janet Katz

What makes a community-based participatory research (CBPR) study successful? This question gets answered whether it is explicitly asked or not. CBPR depends on strong partnerships that can vary in complexity and difficulty, thus making or breaking a project's success. In this way, the question about partnership success is answered in the success of the project. In addition, the meaning of success is flexible and co-created among partners. Some groups of people are especially suspicious, cautious, wary, and dismissive of university researchers. American Indian and Alaska Native (AI/AN) people, because of a long history of exploitation, may be among these. CBPR is not a method but an approach to research. It is an approach that can be responsive to communities who insist on equal power relationships and work that benefits their people, not just the researcher or university. The principles of CBPR—a democratic, community-centered, capacity building and action-oriented process for positive change—make it a good fit for communities. CBPR focuses on strengths instead of just problems. It includes the building of relationships and trust leading to co-learning between partners. CBPR is about increasing community capacity through learning about research and grant writing and increasing university capacity by learning about culture and new strategies for solving persistent problems and health disparities.

The purpose of this chapter is not to provide definitive answers about forming successful partnerships or how to run a research project in indigenous populations; rather, it is to share one study that, in the spirit of inquiry, can be informative and useful by interpreting and understanding others' choices and experiences. It is the recounting of a project that led to a success-ful National Institutes of Health grant application that is being carried out today. A note on terms—we use Native American most frequently to refer to indigenous people of North America because our partners in the Northwest United States use it most often.

BACKGROUND

This initial study was unfunded and the result of a workshop taken at the University of California, Los Angeles (UCLA) School of Nursing on CBPR in 2008. At that time, finding grant funding for a CBPR study was practically nonexistent, especially if the researchers and the community partners had not yet decided on what problems to address or, more to the point, what project or intervention they wanted to do. Our group of unfunded researchers began with two university partners and a community nurse wanting to improve health among the youth in a small AI rural community. We all had ideas of what needed to be done to improve the health of the community, but we did not know what the members of the community wanted. On the advice of the UCLA CBPR mentor, Nancy Anderson, PhD, RN, FAAN, and now professor emerita, we decided to conduct focus groups to understand the community's perspective on the health priorities and needs of their youth.

DESIGN

We chose focus groups as the method and descriptive qualitative research as the methodology to obtain information from a large number of people rep-resenting various constituencies (e.g., elders, youth, geographical location of residence on the reservation, professions) and to capitalize on the inter-actions among members, which ultimately leads to deeper understanding (Morgan, 1997). We used a descriptive qualitative approach with interpre-tation of events and descriptions of experiences. In using descriptive qual-itative research, we did not intend to infer meaning, preferring instead to summarize accurately participants' views (Sandelowski, 2000). In short, we chose a method that would gain the most information in a short time. We were looking for content, that is, opinions; thus we were able to use a descriptive approach. Had we needed more in-depth knowledge or under-standing, we may have chosen an alternative method such as a phenomeno-logical interpretive approach, which is deeply rooted in various philosophical traditions or camps and not appropriate for our purpose described here. Descriptive research may be considered a generic approach because it does not fit any one philosophical tradition. Disadvantages to using a so-called descriptive qualitative method can include establishing rigor.

CONCEPTUAL AND PRACTICAL CONSIDERATIONS

Obtaining Diverse Representation

Because this study was centered on gaining information to guide future work, the main concern was reaching people within the community who represented a wide range of opinions and experiences. Therefore, the most important concern was getting people involved. In any small community, people may be wary of strangers, but in this community, that caution was especially high because of past experiences with non-Native people. As university researchers we were the outsiders. Community members were likely to see us coming to them to "get" without "giving," or as university careerists wanting to advance ourselves without respecting their community or their culture (Jernigan, 2009; Quigley, 2006). Without prior relationships with the community, this study would never have been conducted in the short 2-month timeframe and with the representation as seen in Table 8.1. The partnership between the nurse and the academics was critical in this case.

Tribal and University Institutional Review Board (IRB)

Another concern was obtaining permission from the tribe to conduct our study. As a sovereign nation, an AI or AN tribe sets its own standards for research. These can coincide with the Indian Health Service, with a regional group, or remain solely under their purview. Institutional review was obtained from the university and discussed with the Tribal Council. In this

Table 8.1 *Demographics of Focus Group (%)*

Gender (%)	Age Range (%)		Tribal Membership (%)
Male 37	11–18	25	Member of the tribe 51
Female 63	19–45	25	Other tribe member 25
	46–65	32	Descendent 0.3
	66–100	18	Non-Indian 24
			Live on reservation 97

case, we were able to meet with the Tribal Council and obtain a resolution giving us permission to conduct the focus groups and report findings back to them. Again, prior relationships with tribal members facilitated this process by getting our project on the agenda in a short amount of time.

Before we conducted the focus groups, we met with key stakeholders in the community including teachers and counselors, substance abuse and mental health counselors, and others involved in groups working on youth and community health activities. We discussed ideas and, with their permission and assistance, began brainstorming ways to conduct the focus groups. The stakeholders helped contact people, schedule meetings, and arrange transportation if needed for elders. It cannot be stressed enough that, without this process and partnership, our project would not have occurred as quickly and effectively as it did. To reiterate, CBPR is about relationships and partnership.

Privacy and Confidentiality

A major consideration in research with any community, especially a small community, is privacy and confidentiality. Privacy is related to a participant's volunteering to be in the study or wanting to be left alone. It includes the participant's ability to withhold information he or she does not want to make public. Confidentiality is the trust and right of the individual that information will not be shared without his or her permission. Confidentiality includes giving permission, or not, for the information participants release to be used in public, such as in presentations or publications. Measures to protect participants include conducting interviews in private and de-identification of data through removal of names and any descriptive information that can be used to tell who was talking—including mention of where they live, who their relatives are, and jobs or other social affiliation. Personal identifiers are easy to overlook.

We knew that in a focus group, privacy within the group would be breached if any of the participants discussed personal concerns. Each focus group began with discussion of privacy, and all participants, in their consent form and verbally, were assured that they did not have to participate in the group or discuss anything they did not want to. Focus group members often told us they realized what they said in the group could get to others but agreed not to share private information revealed in the groups. Of course, there is no way to guarantee that; so it was also emphasized to participants that they should not share things they did not want public. To further ensure confidentiality, names and other identifying information were removed from the verbatim transcripts (transcribed from recordings by a professional and human subjects–trained transcriptionist). We did not need to keep track of who said what; so we did not code transcripts other than to know the demographics of the group (for example, an elder group).

Cultural Safety and Sensitivity

A concern in conducting this study was working with people who had, since the colonization of the Americas, experienced ongoing infringement of their rights. For this reason, we considered Native American participants sensitive. In addition, the health topics about tribal youth were sensitive in themselves. For instance, minors' mental health issues, such as suicide, are a sensitive topic. Sensitive, according to Renzetti and Lee (1993), means that the researchers are responsible for looking at the consequences and implications of their work. Renzetti and Lee (1993) define sensitive in terms of the potential threat, or cost, to the participant's psyche and may include emotions such as guilt. A sensitive topic is "one that potentially poses for those involved a substantial threat, the emergence of which renders problematic for the researcher and/or the researched collection, holding, and/or dissemination of research data" (Renzetti & Lee, 1993, p. 5). This study attempted to offer protection through avoiding unnecessary intrusions of privacy and ensuring confidentiality. In addition, community partners were asked before the focus groups to assess potential harm and community benefit (Katz, 2005). Community benefit was identified as reducing health disparities, identification of a health issue supported by the community as a priority, and writing a grant for potential funding to address the priority. No harm was identified.

Cultural safety, unlike cultural competency, is defined from the perspective of the person or community. The term cultural safety came from Aotero, New Zealand, when indigenous Maori and nonindigenous New Zealanders were working together (Doutrich et al., 2012). It is based on critical theory that calls on researchers and partners to take societal class and power, disenfranchisement, and oppression into consideration for a project. In our project, as well as others in the United States, the concept of cultural safety is an integral part of working together that goes both ways. The question we ask ourselves as partners is: Do I feel respected and safe? You have to be able to talk to each other to discover the answers to this question. This is an ongoing process that takes time and, again, relationship. Cultural safety is a concept that many indigenous researchers say must be understood and practiced (Papps & Ramsden, 1996).

Culture and Tribes

There are no cultural rules or guidelines that fit all Native Americans or other indigenous people, but some general ideas may hold true. Showing respect is done by deferring to elders, serving food, and, in some cases, giving gifts. This project's community partners helped the university partners understand the cultural norms and how to be culturally appropriate in showing respect and appreciation. Because we were meeting with many elders, we often joined them for lunch at the senior centers and gave them small gifts of appreciation. Further, we met with youth at places convenient to them, such as schools and youth centers. For employees of the tribe or schools, we went to their workplaces and met them at lunch or after work. Essentially, we did whatever was needed to make focus group participation convenient and appropriate. Many Native American academics and communities identify CBPR as culturally appropriate, so the choice to use CPBR as a research approach in this instance was fitting and culturally respectful.

DATA ANALYSIS

Preparation for Data Analysis

Data analysis was conducted with our partners and through the formation of a community advisory board (CAB). At each focus group, we asked people to volunteer for the CAB. The purpose of the CAB was to help analyze data to determine the community's priority for the health of its youth, to consider what types of projects could help, and to assist in writing a grant to obtain project funding. Of the 25 volunteers, 12 members, many of whom worked with youth in the youth centers or schools, participated in the CAB meetings. At the first meeting we conducted human subject training. There are many ways to do this, and we suggest searching for a method that works for your community. A great deal has been written on this topic in the last few years. Considerations include how computer savvy CAB members are, the degree (or amount) of information they wish to know, and decisions on best ways to present.

Another important topic to cover is describing what CBPR is. This can vary depending on the group and its wishes. We chose an abbreviated session because the CAB members stated they did not want to spend time on it. Other Native American researchers have reported they do not do CBPR training because Native people are very familiar with working together in this way.

Data Analysis as an Iterative Process

The focus group digital recordings were transcribed and identifiers removed. The university partners listened to all the recordings and used field notes taken during the focus groups to clarify any inaudible or recording difficulties. An in-depth summary of the transcripts, which incorporated key elements of the focus groups along with quotes, was developed and taken to the first CAB meeting for members to read and discuss (Morgan, 1997; Rabiee, 2004; Webb & Kevern, 2000). We also provided information about human subjects' rights and CBPR information along with introductions over a meal. After this meeting, the university partners met and reread the transcripts and the CAB's outline of themes. University partners met again and compared findings and resolved any differences they had through discussions. At the second CAB meeting, themes were reviewed and consensus reached. The CAB discussed the priority community concerns identified in the focus groups. The CAB was asked to identify questions they wanted to explore further—research questions and aims for the grant writing—and what kinds of projects they wanted to pursue. In hindsight, the researchers realized they were expecting CAB members to already understand, or have interest in, thinking about research questions and thus, be able to help formulate specific questions. However, CAB members were not interested in formulating questions; rather, they were interested in coming up with projects to solve concerns and problems. This situation frustrated researchers who were naïve and going by "the book." So, lessons learned included taking the lead of community members to meet their needs and to work on co-education if so desired. Such a lesson serves as an example of what building capacity on both sides of the partnership represents.

Rigor

We maintained rigor throughout our iterative process, in part to take into consideration varying viewpoints on the data and in part to alleviate bias when possible. In addition, we kept notes during the focus groups and during university and CAB meetings to create documentation that could be referred to if needed. The CAB gave insider perspectives about the data and in the analysis to help reduce research bias and to verify truthfulness of findings. To clarify, in quantitative research, rigor refers to validity or truthfulness of the findings, while reliability refers to the stability of the findings or how much variation is present. In qualitative research, the following concepts are important to understand: (a) truthfulness or confirmability—how well do findings represent what participants said (can be judged by participants themselves) versus the researchers' preconceived ideas or biases?; (b) dependability—how does analysis fit findings (demonstrated if needed by keeping close track of the process through field notes)?; and (c) transferability— how can findings be used to understand other situations (Katz, Oneal, & Paul, 2011)? There are other definitions and concepts related to rigor in qualitative research that include creativity and integrity, not to mention practicality of application (Whittemore, Chase, & Mandle, 2001). The overall purpose is to make sure the participants' voices are represented and respected.

RESULTS

There were 13 focus groups consisting of 95 participants ranging in age from 11 to 99. The majority of participants were tribal members. Others were members of other tribes, or non-Natives. Most participants lived on the reservation. The results clearly pointed to substance use and mental health issues, such as suicide and unresolved grief, as the primary community concerns for their youth (Katz, Martinez, & Paul, 2011).

After the focus group study, university and community partners applied for three grants from the Centers for Disease Control and Prevention (CDC), U.S. Department of Agriculture (USDA), and Agency for Healthcare Research and Quality (AHRQ). None were funded. In 2013, we applied for a CBPR grant from the National Institute for Minority Health and received funding. At present we have a resolution from the tribe to proceed. We met with our CAB and held a kick-off event that included a lunch, presentations, and discussions with the 40 participants. Challenges have included changes in tribal personnel, proceeding with budgeting through subcontracts, and meetings made difficult because of varying schedules, distances, cellphone reception, and, at times, Internet connections. The focus of our grant is to develop a pilot project to address the results of the 2008 focus group results reported in this chapter. We plan to begin the pilot project early in 2015.

DISSEMINATION

Dissemination began with writing up results and sharing with the Tribal Council. We also wrote a short article that went into the local newspaper. Because of time constraints at the time, we did not host a community meeting although this would have been a very good idea. In addition, we should have continued to have meetings to stay visible in the community. The Tribal

Council has changed members, so those we worked with initially are currently not in office. We should have continued to have regular meetings with council members as new members came in. As noted in the introduction, you find out what makes a project a success without even asking, and even if you ask, you find things you did not expect. The key is observing and reflecting.

A paper was written with partners and was published in 2008. In addition, this work was presented at the Transcultural Nursing Conference and in a poster at two university symposia. Continued dissemination includes our current work. We shared the focus group process and results at community meetings, the kickoff event, Tribal Council meetings, and CAB meetings.

SUMMARY

This study's importance to our current work has been critical. Without previous relationships in place with community partners, the study described here could not have been completed nor could the current pilot project have begun. Crucial to the success of a study such as this is the ongoing relationship between both parties. Forming and nurturing relationships takes time and effort, an aspect of CBPR that could be overlooked or minimized if unfamiliar with the approach. Choosing CBPR to address adolescent health in a Native American community has been challenging and rewarding but, in the end, is one of the few approaches that respectfully and sensitively includes all partners.

REFERENCES

Doutrich, D., Arcus, K., Dekker, L., Spuck, J., & Pollock-Robinson, C. (2012). Cultural safety in New Zealand and the United States: Looking at a way forward together. *Journal of Transcultural Nursing, 23*(2), 143–150.

Jernigan, V. B. B. (2009). Community-based participatory research with Native American communities: The chronic disease self-management program. *Health Promotion Practice, 11*(6), 888–899.

Katz, J. (2005). "If I could do it they could do it:" A collective case study of plateau tribes' nurses. *Journal of American Indian Education, 44*(2), 36–51.

Katz, J. R., Martinez, T. A., & Paul, R. (2011). Community based participatory research and American Indian Alaska native nurse practitioners: A partnership to promote adolescent health. *Journal of American Academy of Nurse Practitioners, 23*, 298–304.

Katz, J. R., Oneal, G., & Paul, R. (2011). "I don't know if I can make it": Native American students considering college and career. *Online Journal of Cultural Competence in Nursing and Healthcare, 1*(4), 11–26.

Morgan, D. L. (1997). *Focus groups as qualitative research.* Thousand Oaks, CA: Sage.

Papps, E., & Ramsden, I. (1996). Cultural safety in nursing: The New Zealand experience. *International Journal for Quality in Health Care, 8*(5), 491–497.

Quigley, D. (2006). A review of improved ethical practices in environmental and public health research: Case examples from native communities. *Health Education and Behavior, 30*(2), 130–147.

Rabiee, F. (2004). Focus group and data analysis. *Proceedings of the Nutrition Society, 63*, 655–660.

Renzetti, C. M., & Lee, R. M. (1993). *Researching sensitive topics.* Newbury Park, CA: Sage.

Sandelowski, M. (2000). Whatever happened to qualitative description. *Research in Nursing & Health, 23*, 334–340.

Webb, C., & Kevern, J. (2000). Focus group as a research method: A critique of some aspects of their use in nursing research. *Journal of Advanced Nursing, 33*(6), 798–805.

Whittemore, R., Chase, S. K., & Mandle, C. L. (2001). Validity in qualitative research. *Qualitative Health Research, 11*(4), 522–537.

CHAPTER NINE

HOW TO CONDUCT PARTICIPATORY ACTION RESEARCH: AN EXEMPLAR

Lorna Kendrick

PARTICIPATORY ACTION RESEARCH AS TRADITION

According to Glasson and colleagues (2008), participatory action research (PAR) is cyclical and involves moving from reflection, planning, action, and observation, then back to reflection to repeat the process with the goal being to bring about change. Yet others describe participation, action, and inquiry as the heart of PAR. Regardless of which definition is used, the terms *transformation* and *empowerment* tend to undergird the ideology of researchers and their studies when PAR is used to guide the design. The terms transformation and empowerment bring to mind words such as *change, strengthen, new, growth, alter,* or *liberate.* As such, the purpose of PAR for all who choose to conduct this type of research is more than understanding phenomena; it is transforming and/or empowering all those involved, from researchers to study participants.

When we think about the tradition of research from a historic perspective, we recognize the primary goals were to gain an understanding of phenomena as well as discover how phenomena are interconnected or related to one another. In the human quest to explain and understand our world, we use research to peer into the complexity of phenomena from as many vantage points as is possible. We not only discover the interconnectedness of phenomena but also the reasons why some phenomena exist as well as ways to improve and change phenomena for the benefit of humankind.

Research Tradition/History Influencing My Study

Historically, the only way to discover truth about phenomena was the process of being guided by a positivist worldview to gain as true and complete an understanding as possible. This positivist worldview was typically steeped in logic, statistics, and manipulation of variables.

The positivist worldview provided a strong scientific systematic process recognized the world over as a trusted method to discover truth with few errors. However, as the nation began to shift, becoming more culturally diverse, many research findings were questioned as to the accuracy and validity of data when applied to diverse groups. In response, there were processes for reconfiguring philosophy, ideology, standards, beliefs, and values resulting in developments such as the women's and minority rights movements. Through these processes, many "norms" were challenged and retooled, ushering in reformation and new respect for diversity in the ways of knowing and in many aspects of life and thinking. This reformation also influenced the traditions used to guide the directions, methods, and designs for research from this point on.

This was a strategic and exciting time for many researchers wanting to step beyond a generalizable understanding of phenomena alone. This transitional time in history also brought with it changes in who could and would choose a research career. With the changing and evolving look, attitudes, and beliefs of persons entering research as well as their diversity in training, research projects were also moving in new and innovative directions.

Of those choosing research careers, many were young, with new ideas and areas of interest based on their own lived experiences. In addition to changes in researchers, there were often more diverse groups being represented as human subjects (e.g., women, culturally diverse groups, etc.), hence generating an increasing need for alternate methods to engage and recruit participants to represent the changing needs and faces of our nation.

This convergence of a number of historic and societal factors resulted in a kind of awakening within all areas of learning, resulting in a naturally occurring evolution of thought, particularly among researchers new to the field. With this evolution came the personal experiences of the newer researchers from which they began designing studies. Many of their concerns were related to inequities and marginalization they may have experienced prior to their tenure as researchers. Many of today's research mentors often share these experiences and stories positing how these factors led to their often amazing findings and opportunities as seasoned experts in their fields of research.

PAR was a natural byproduct of this convergence of factors at a time in history primed and ready for a paradigm shift. This paradigm shift readiness was especially noted in society during the 1950s and 1960s when the nation began to witness people (e.g., women and minority groups) risking life and limb to make their demands for change known. Not only were we forced as a nation into an awareness of human inequities close to home, but we were also forced to witness the destruction and devastations of war. This first-hand exposure through the nightly news in our homes via television seemed to impart an attitude of concern to our society that had been easily lost with the anonymity of words written in a newspaper. Instead, we were introduced to real people experiencing inequities in our nation and the devastations of war around the world.

With increasing awareness and concern as a nation, we witnessed growth in volunteerism and service. For many, the focus on service to community further strengthened their respect and value for others, leading to a need and desire to better understand the life experiences of others. With this, researchers were motivated to use their knowledge, understanding, and training (e.g., systematic inquiry) to begin the process of understanding the life experiences of others to empower and transform their lives.

For example, the purpose of our study was to begin to understand and describe perceptions of depression (Kendrick, 2003). In addition to gaining a better understanding as researchers, our participants described feelings of relief after sharing their stories. The young men also expressed a desire to share with others, so they too would feel the "emotional strength" they developed as a result of finding others in the group discussions with similar life experiences.

CONCEPTUALIZATION PHASE: DECIDING TO USE PAR

Our study employed both ethnography and PAR for design, method, data collection, data analysis, and dissemination of findings to empower, transform, and understand the perceptions of young African American men about depression and their mental health. Ethnography as a tradition focuses on understanding what captivates a cultural group through immersing one's self in the participants' or groups' daily lives and world.

PAR was the perfect complementary process to combine with ethnography to delve into an understanding of the perceptions of young African American men. The challenges associated with being an African American male and the ongoing struggles among this group to transform society's assumptions about them and find empowerment through this process demanded the use of PAR to allow them to tell their stories of perceptions through research.

Why PAR?

What motivated this study was a desire to make a difference in the lives of young African American men. I was often frustrated by stories on the nightly news reporting on a small percentage of African American men who had chosen to take from rather than contribute to society as representing the entirety of African American men. Rarely did I see African American men represented on the nightly news as most of the ones I knew, who were contributing to society positively, caring for their families, and making positive choices. I was saddened knowing most Americans would continue to judge these young men by the worst of society being represented on the nightly news and in our written media.

Additionally, as culturally diverse researchers reading published data findings on African Americans, my colleagues and I would often wonder who the participants were, because few findings represented anyone we knew. We noted data were most often collected from participants living within the confines of poverty, not in our opinion representative of the diversity among African Americans. For example a young African American male participant from our study made the following statement:

> I wonder how would they feel if we called them all trailer trash, so why do they think they can judge us all by stereotypes and assumptions and what they see on TV or the news. I have never been in trouble, but they are scared of me just because I'm young, male, and African American. ... People are not all the same, just like them, we are all different. ... I am not a thug, my grandparents were not poor, my parents were not poor, I am not poor, and I am not violent, I don't steal, I have a job, I went to college. ... Can you believe a lady locked her car door when she saw me pull up next to her, like I wanted her 1988 Toyota, and I'm driving a 2010 Infinity I got by working hard, give me a break. ...

My desire was to recruit a more affluent group of African Americans for my research and begin to see if in fact the data would hold up when we looked at a variety of people and not just the poor. It was at this point I began conversations with people in my community.

However, I must digress and share an experience I had a few months before I began my discussions with community members and young men. As a doctoral student working as a research assistant, I had an interesting encounter that changed me as a future researcher. A clinic director said to me, "I will share this with you because I think you will understand and be able to explain it to those you work with; I am not going to give these researchers any more names. This community is tired of university people coming in and taking data for their own professional success. They benefit from our stories but give us nothing in return."

I have never been the same since this conversation. I have always been truly grateful to this director for taking the time to share this with me. Too often in life, we instinctively have concerns but often believe the concerns are probably our own fears and limitations, thus convincing ourselves to move on. However, in this case the clinic director validated a deeply intuitive concern I had but did not know how to define or address it until she shared her thoughts and concerns. This encounter awakened and stirred a deeper understanding within me of my own fundamental values, philosophy, and ideology that I needed to hold on to so my research would not lose contextual truth.

Recognizing and becoming comfortable with this reality of self was necessary in my personal and professional transformation as a future researcher. This encounter and self-discovery propelled and motivated me to search for a philosophy of research I could use to honor the participants, their life stories, and experiences within the data we were collecting. These experiences within my own life story led to the beginning of PAR as foundational to my worldview as a researcher.

The following statement by a participant, in response to a question posed by a researcher in the audience during a research conference where we were presenting our data findings, deepened my commitment and motivation and further confirmed that the use of PAR with diverse groups is compulsory and a fundamental right. This is a poignant example of why PAR methods were employed to design, collect, and analyze data as well as disseminate our findings. The young man put it this way,

> Research is typically designed based on your thoughts and ideas. When we the participants say to you none of the responses fit my reality, you the researchers say just choose the one option that comes closest to your thinking ... you say this even though I have already told you none fit. This tells me you don't care about my truth; you only want to validate your own truth. So for me, the participatory research method showed respect for me, my thoughts, and who I am as a person; it caused me to want to tell my story. Not only did I answer questions, I had input on what types of questions or responses were used to even get at my truth. How can you design research about me when you don't even know me and don't seem to want to know me? Truth in your mind is still based on your assumptions about things. If my truth challenges your assumptions, you don't want to hear it. So for the sake of "science," you hide behind your research design, rarely discovering truth. So guess what, I am not going to tell you my story. Instead I will respond with

the answers your attitude tells me you expect to hear. So now I know your research findings are all based on what you want or expect to hear. So when you say African American men have more this or that, I don't buy it 'cause I know you searched for and got what you were looking for, a lie. But I can tell you this for a fact, this research about how we feel about depression is the truth, and any guy of color born in America will tell you this is his story too. But of course you say qualitative research cannot be generalized, but I say if you do it right, it actually can. It still amazes me how many guys, both African American and Latino, say "wow that's so true" when they read the article we wrote.

MY STUDY AS AN EXEMPLAR

Design Issues

The purpose of this study was to describe the perceptions and experiences of young African American men about depression and feelings and thoughts of despair. This qualitative study was a combination of ethnographic methods, such as participant observation, group discussions, and individual interviews, combined with PAR methods, such as community partnerships and networking, used with African American young men in community-based settings to discover their views about depression and feelings of despair. The participants included 28 young African American men 18 to 25 years of age.

This study was conducted in two phases. During Phase One, 20 African American young men 18 to 25 years of age were recruited for participation in five group discussions. During Phase Two, I met frequently with several of the Phase One participants to conduct individual interviews and additional group discussions to clarify emerging categories as well as check the accuracy of participant observations described in my field notes. During Phase Two, 8 newly recruited young men participated in additional individual interviews and group discussions. The purpose of meeting with the newly recruited young men was to verify emerging categories as well as check for any additional categories that might emerge; however, no new information or categories emerged.

As I was developing my research proposal, I spent many hours talking with members of the community discussing thoughts and ideas for this study. In particular there was one young man who began as an expert "guide" sharing his thoughts and ideas, but later joined the study team when we struggled with recruitment. I spent hours with this young man and many of his African American male friends. Together we attended concerts and movies, played basketball, and listened to music. I "hung out" with them observing their interactions, language, choice of clothing, and listening intently as they discussed school, women, politics, and their feelings about being African American men.

The young men from the community introduced me to other young men, not their close friends, but young men they typically only interacted with in such places as the basketball court or their college or university campus cafeteria. These young men on the outer fringes of our research relationship were also very receptive to me because I was with the young men who had become my community network, and they were also willing to discuss their ideas about a study on the perceptions of young African American men.

I also spent many hours discussing my ideas with my African American friends and colleagues. Everyone I discussed my ideas with was excited and always willing to offer names of other people in the community they thought could be of help to me. Each person I discussed my ideas with wanted to offer suggestions on, for example, "what questions I should ask" or "what groups of young men I should focus on" during the study.

During one such conversation with a friend, the suggestion was made that I consider their church as a possible place to both glean ideas and recruit participants. The suggestion was made because the church membership of approximately 2,800 included a larger number of African Americans and was very involved in working with youth. Many of the church programs were focused on young African American men. It was also noted their associate pastor was about the same age as the young men I was planning to recruit.

The youth pastor was very helpful making suggestions about how to approach the young men in their church. He shared experiences from his own life and observations from interactions with his college friends and church community. He offered ideas for questions and approaches that might increase the receptiveness of the young men. The youth pastor also had ideas about what members might be good key informants. Prior to the suggestion by my friend and contacting the youth pastor, I had visited the church on several occasions. Following my discussions with the pastor, each time I visited the church I was more observant of the environment. I watched the young men and noted such things as their interactions, behavior, choice of clothing, and language.

I was introduced to the church community by the senior pastor during a regular worship service. The youth pastor introduced me to several key church members at different points during the months when we

were developing a partnership for this project. These members were identified as potentially interested and willing to work with me during the final
development phases of the project. Prior to this introductory process, the
youth pastor briefed these members and described my interest in how young
African American men describe depression.

It was through these key church members that many of my participants
were recruited. From these conversations as well as the conversations with the
young man in my community network, his friends, my friends and colleagues,
and the youth pastor, I gathered valuable suggestions and ideas for this study.
This community participation was strategic to the success of this study.

Church and community members openly discussed my research ideas
and asked many clarifying questions. They asked me for more information
about the kind of young men I wanted to talk to. They also wanted me to
clarify my goals. They wanted to make sure I was concerned about the welfare
of potential participants. Some of their questions addressed concerns such as
"What are you planning to do with the data?" and "How will participants/
the community benefit from your research?"

To build rapport and become more a part of these communities,
I attended weekly church services as well as other community activities that
the young men frequented. I also spent time on their college campuses discussing my thoughts and ideas, meeting and discussing the potential study
with their college counselors and advisors as well as observing their daily
lives and routines.

The church has a full calendar of events each week that includes activities
such as choir rehearsals, singles meetings, community counseling services,
community outreach, bowling nights, prayer meetings, and co-ed volleyball.
The community services offered serve as both church-wide functions as well
as individual church member functions. For example, one member, also a
member of our community network, works with inner-city youth providing
job training, counseling, and mentorship. I spent time talking with him,
observing activities involved in the training program as well as meeting and
talking to many of the program participants.

Another example of a community activity was a "jazz under the stars"
musical concert on the church grounds. I attended the concert with church
and community members, several of the pastors from local churches, and an
array of residents from several surrounding communities. After attending a
variety of community activities, most members began to call me by name,
chose me to be on their teams during activities, invited me to other social functions not associated with church activities, and talked about their personal
lives and their beliefs. My research also became a topic of conversation
during many of these activities.

After approximately a year spent immersing myself within these community networks, I developed my research design incorporating their suggestions and ideas. My research methods, procedures, and data collection were also developed with the thoughts and ideas shared by the community interspersed throughout.

Once the design, methods, procedures, and data collection were completed, I took this information back to members of the community for review. I sent out e-mail invitations and posted invitations at the church and in their college campus dorms, asking community members to attend a meeting where I would share the proposed research design with them. This time of review with the community was used to both impart information about as well as seek consensus and support for the design. The evening I presented the design to the community, the discussion included questions as well as clarification of terms. Once I received support from the community for the research design, I submitted the study proposal to the institutional review board (IRB).

The first step in data collection was to conduct five group discussions. During the group discussions PAR was experienced at its best when the members decided who among them would facilitate the group discussion. Instead of the researcher leading the groups, the young men led the group discussions for all group meetings. The young men suggested selecting alternate names for each group member to ensure their identities would be protected during the tape recorded discussion. Thus each young man decided upon a name for himself. A couple of the participants struggled, and the other men suggested a name based on the color of a shirt or what may have been written on this shirt.

I offered the young men the choice of having a copy of the interview questions. The groups decided they wanted to have a copy of the questions and determined they would answer the questions by going around the table in their seating order. Each young man offered an answer to each question. No one asked to be skipped. When the young man seated next to him completed his answer, the next young man automatically began his turn.

The following is an excerpt from my field notes describing my reaction to the first group discussion:

Wow this was so exciting. ... I never thought about having the young men facilitate the group discussions. I am so happy they volunteered (wow they even had someone in charge of changing the tape, how funny they made everyone be quiet while they changed the tape so they wouldn't lose any "data"). ... I think it made such a difference having them read the questions and put their own spin on the words and explanation of questions (I stayed quiet and let them figure it out). When they struggled to figure out the gist of the question, I am glad they (not me) made the determination what the meaning was.... This kept my thoughts and ideas out of it.... I think if I would have been facilitating, "I" would have gotten in the way somehow.... This is also good because it reduces the likelihood of me influencing their thoughts and responses ... this was such a great discussion, there were times they would all talk at the same time when they were excited or agreed about something being said. **Note I stopped them at 90 minutes and reminded them they signed the consent for a 90 minutes group discussion and they were not required to stay longer.... They all stated they wanted to continue ... this group went 3 hours and 40 minutes.... I better inform the IRB just in case.... Wow!!! This was so cool; I could never have imagined my very first group would go so smoothly and so exceptionally well.... It seemed like a catharsis for them.... They shared so much and didn't want to stop talking. About 4 of them (Mr. Blue, Mr. Green, Mr. Orange, and Mr. Yellow) said they felt like a weight had been lifted off their shoulders talking about all this stuff....

After the group discussions and individual interviews were completed and transcribed, I began my data analysis process. I reviewed tapes again while rereading transcriptions to ensure accuracy. After reviewing the transcripts for accuracy I was able to do the analysis of data by identifying and tabulating repeated topics from the transcribed data. I coded repeated topics using a color-coded dot system. I then combined these repeated topics into logical data clusters.

Once data clusters were developed, I shared these data with the study participants. Sharing the data findings (an aspect of PAR) offered the participants an opportunity to provide consensus and clarify their data. By involving the participants in clarifying the data, I was able to avoid many potential coding errors that may have been missed if I alone had interpreted the statements made by the young men. After sharing the categories from the data with study participants, I reexamined the clusters of the categories in relationship to the participants' comments and the field note data recorded on the participant observation templates to organize the findings into stronger cluster groups. It was from these cluster groups that the participants and I formed the final categories and appropriate data-based conclusions. On three separate occasions, members of my professional advisory board also looked at the data providing their professional thoughts and ideas about the process rather than the content.

Challenges

The first challenge I faced was my topic. None of the young men walking by my poster wanted to discuss "depression." One man, who appeared older than 18 to 25, responded, "Why don't you talk about prostate cancer? You would get a lot more men who would talk to you about that, but I doubt anyone will ever volunteer to talk about depression."

At the time my youngest son was between 18 to 25 years of age. Each week during our family walks, we would discuss my research ideas. My son would provide me with very helpful and insightful thoughts and ideas related to working with young men of his generation and ethnicity. Hence, when we discussed my first recruitment challenges, it was my son who suggested someone who looked like the potential participants would be much more effective in recruiting. At which time he volunteered to help with recruitment. I was concerned the IRB would not allow my son to recruit participants for a study I was conducting.

I was pleasantly surprised when the IRB approved having my son assist with recruitment and other aspects of the study. As my son suggested, he effortlessly recruited the first eight participants by simply telling them about the study topic. From this point on, the newest participants recruited became the recruitment team for the next group of participants. As such, the first 20 participants were recruited through a snowball recruitment method. The final eight participants were recruited through a community contact at a university about 100 miles away.

The snowball recruitment we used was not based on recruiting friends exclusively, but other college students not always known by participants were stopped on campus and asked if they would be interested in participating in group discussions about their perceptions of depression. Additionally, a couple of the college students who attended the community church and were involved in design discussions participated in group meetings. This also opened recruitment to young men who were not all friends or friends of friends. I believe this snowball method was more efficient because it opened recruitment to more than just friends and close associates, which could result in participants with very similar or the same life experiences.

Another challenge I was concerned about and wanted to carefully build in safety factors to address was the protection of the truth of the data against any potential biases on my part as an African American woman. There was the potential risk I would become more sensitive than objective and analytic to the young men's stories. Hence, I had a professional advisory board to work with who carefully reviewed design, procedures, group discussion transcripts, fieldnotes, and so on throughout the process to ensure I (as well as the participants and community members) stayed true to the design and did not go "native" or lose my ability to remain an impartial observer.

Rigor

As a proponent of PAR and with a desire to transform and empower these young men, it was important to me that the data were as accurate and truthful as possible. Therefore, credibility, consistency, and neutrality were used to establish rigorous guidelines and boundaries for this study as well as decrease the likelihood of any unexpected risks occurring. PAR and ethnography provided a triangulation of methods allowing me to verify data from one method with data from another method (e.g., interview data with observations).

Study credibility or truth-value was strengthened through both the PAR process in designing the study and the participants' own statements about their feelings and beliefs. Additionally, the PAR model gave the participants the opportunity to review and validate their truths when they were asked to substantiate their statements. Consistency or repeatability was enhanced by developing and describing in detail the research design and methodology.

Finally, neutrality was used to decrease the risk of bias. Keeping neutrality in mind, I maintained awareness of appropriate professional boundaries and objectivity by being actively supervised by colleagues on my professional advisory board throughout the research process and, in particular, during the data collection and analysis process. The research methodology was carefully designed to provide specific guidelines such as field notes describing my feelings and responses to the environment, participant and community feedback at all phases, and audit trails to describe how and why certain data analysis decisions were made.

As an American of African descent myself, neutrality was especially important to decrease the likelihood of my own personal biases, ideas, and experiences from influencing the collection, interpretation, and analysis of data. Additionally, the PAR design included methodological processes to allow participants to guide and direct the individual interviews and group discussions. Using an open-ended, blank slate type of interview procedure helped to decrease the risk of participants' becoming biased by ideas generated from a more structured researcher-designed pool of questions.

A very interesting and unexpected challenge presented itself when my son shared an impactful encounter with the police during a group discussion. At that moment I had to make a decision—"mom or researcher." I chose to uphold the confidentiality of consent and the rigor of my design and remained the objective researcher. Later during our debriefing with my son and the second facilitator, my son volunteered his thoughts and reasoning for this sharing (noted in my field notes). He said he shared his story both because it was appropriate at the moment and it also showed his comfort with sharing in my presence, helping to break the ice for other participants.

Later when I analyzed these data I was initially concerned he may have unduly influenced the others by attempting "to show them they could trust me." However, I noted the group discussion participants had already been sharing openly and without hesitation, and in subsequent group discussions, I noted other newly recruited facilitators using similar "build rapport with researcher in the room" tactics. When I took the data back to the participants for member-checking, I actually asked them about this. Each group discussion participant who acted as facilitator shared that this was a process they typically use when there's an older person present who they want their friends to know is safe and can be trusted. It was a naturally occurring part of their group norm.

How Did I Resolve Problems?

Interestingly there were few noted problems. I believe this was directly related to the PAR model being used throughout the study. The inclusion of members of the lay community in planning and idea-generating discussions seemed to result in any potential problems being addressed during those discussions. As mentioned earlier, upon hearing my challenges with recruitment, my son volunteered to assist. My initial reaction was "the IRB will never allow this." After discussing my son's suggestion with my research mentor, I followed up with the IRB. The benefit of being connected to an IRB with a solid understanding of qualitative design was quickly evident. The IRB agreed to allow my son to act as my "key informant" or "guide" as we chose to use the term.

It was quite interesting to observe the reaction of the young men to my son compared to their reaction to me. Even in alternative sites, using a "guide" of their same gender and ethnicity, although older, helped to make the young men more receptive to participating in a research study where depression was the topic of discussion.

What may seem quite benign, but could easily be considered a problem, was that, when the young men began their group discussions, there was a kind of cathartic affect. The young men had never really had the opportunity or avenue to share these thoughts and ideas, so they were able to release a variety of frustrations and feelings. So much so that the 90-minute group discussion time the IRB had approved was quickly extended. At the 90-minute point, I stopped the discussion and reminded the participants of the 90-minute time frame they agreed to when they signed the informed consent, at which time each young man agreed to continue. Our first group discussion lasted 3 hours 40 minutes; following this group meeting, I returned to the IRB for approval to extend our group discussion times.

Another interesting occurrence happened when I was out in the community "hanging out" with participants, conducting participant observations. The young men were extremely excited to be participating in research where they felt valued and where their lifestories were, in their words, "going to make a difference in their community." So often when we were in public areas (e.g., college, gym, at a game, walking through a mall, etc.), they would call someone they knew over to substantiate their statements. At this point I had to again seek counsel from my research mentor regarding who needed to give consent and who didn't need to give consent.

How Decisions Were Made

I recognized how important it was for me to spend time with the participants after the group discussions as well as time with members of the community prior to the beginning of the data collection. This time I spent—immersing myself in the participants' lives, reviewing my field notes, taking the data back to the participants, recruiting eight new participants to check similarities and/or for any new data, as well as reviewing as audits conducted by my professional advisory board—helped me make decisions during data analysis.

Additionally, reading and rereading data while listening to transcripts, as well as color-coding data myself rather than using qualitative data analysis programs, helped me become extremely familiar with the dataset. This familiarity with the dataset also strengthened my understanding and my ability to connect data within the context of the young men's lives, resulting in trustworthy findings. I didn't really recognize this until I took the data back to the young men for member-checking, at which point they each felt I had really "nailed" their comments well. Furthermore, when data were reviewed by one of the professionals on the advisory board, her analysis of a section of data was congruent with my data analysis findings of the same section of data.

IN REVIEW

I was introduced to and guided through PAR by my dissertation chair, to whom I am exceedingly grateful. However, the participants and the community provided a life-changing richness not found in the literature. Following each group discussion, I would meet with the co-facilitators to "process or debrief" the group discussion experiences. Interestingly, because I spent so much time in the community prior to beginning the research, the young men appeared to be comfortable with me and had a desire to "help" or "guide" me through their world and their stories. They would often define terms for me or further explain a thought. I found that the data collection did not end when the group discussions were over. For example, a young man once turned up the radio and directed me to listen to the words because the words of the song further clarified what was discussed during our previous group meeting.

I have to say I am most proud of our dissemination of the findings. I believe we have taken PAR to a level few have taken it to, but a place it should naturally go to. Not only have some of our participants been coauthors on our articles, but they have also traveled to conferences and presented with us.

Currently, some of the former participants are members of our advisory board, constituted once the research was completed. Whenever we consider further research or review of data, they are included in the discussion. When questions or new ideas are generated from data, the information is shared with the advisory board. When I see any of the young men all these years later, they greet me as if I am their mom, and we reminisce about our experiences as research collaborators and change agents.

The very nature of PAR as we experienced it elicits long-term cooperative partnerships and transformed lives for all involved in the process. The process of participation within PAR runs the gamut of possibilities when the way to involve participants and the community is considered. When one considers research with human subjects, the beliefs, ideals, and values of those participants cannot be discounted. To increase the truth and trustworthiness of data, PAR should always be a serious consideration both in qualitative and quantitative designs.

REFERENCES

Glasson, J. B., Chang, E. M., & Bidewell, J. W. (2008). The value of participatory action research in clinical nursing practice. *International Journal of Nursing Practice*, *14*(1), 34–39.

Kendrick, L. D. (2003). *The views of young African-American men about depression*. University of California, Los Angeles. ProQuest, UMI Dissertations Publishing. (3088990)

CHAPTER TEN

EXPLORING PARENTAL PERCEPTIONS OF HEALTHY EATING AND PHYSICAL ACTIVITY USING THE PHOTOVOICE METHOD

Nicole Mareno

I believe that helping families achieve a healthy lifestyle is an essential nursing action. My area of research focus is prevention and treatment of childhood obesity. The rates of overweight and obesity among children and adolescents in this country are skyrocketing; according to the most current data, 31.7% of 2- to 19-year old children and adolescents now exceed the 85th percentile for body mass index (BMI) for age, with 11.9% of the group exceeding the 95th percentile (Ogden, Curtin, Carroll, Lamb, & Flegal, 2010). High rates of overweight and obesity among children and adolescents are a public health threat. Nurses can assist families to access early, preventive health care and education about modifiable lifestyle behaviors like healthy diets and physical activity.

Health behaviors are learned in the home environment, and children begin to emulate their parents' dietary and physical activity patterns from an early age (Golan & Crow, 2004). Parents are children's primary role models for eating and physical activity, and are the key change agents within the family system. I am going to describe to you a community-based participatory research (CBPR) approach that you can use to gain an understanding about an individual's perception of life and health. In my study, I sought to understand parents' perception of what helped and hindered their family from eating healthy and being physically active. The outcome of this project was a greater understanding of assets and barriers to healthy eating and physical activity. The next step in my program of research is to develop a family-tailored weight management intervention, building on what I learned in this study.

COMMUNITY-BASED PARTICIPATORY RESEARCH

I start by describing the community-based participatory research (CBPR) approach. CBPR engages researchers and community members in a critical dialogue about supportive and detrimental factors impacting health (Olshansky, 2008). The result of this discussion can be used to create interventions tailored directly to the needs of the population or community.

In my study, I used a CBPR approach and employed the photovoice data collection method (Wang & Burris, 1997). Photovoice is a powerful tool for community change that allows individuals to reflect and communicate their everyday life experiences through the use of images captured with a camera. Photovoice is rooted in critical theory (Freire, 1970), with a strong feminist perspective (Wang & Burris, 1997). Freire was a proponent of allowing individuals to document how social forces impact their everyday lives through visual images. In his research, Freire used photographs to encourage community dialogue about social and political issues. Women's voices have often been silenced in research; photovoice empowers women to share their everyday experiences. Weiler (1988) asserts that feminist research methodologies respect and appreciate women's subjective experiences and knowledge. As Wang (1999) notes, researchers can learn how women portray their own lives by handing them a camera.

The main goal of photovoice is to communicate subjective experiences by documenting everyday life with a camera (Wang & Burris, 1997). Armed with a camera, individuals can document social, cultural, and economic conditions that impact their health. Photovoice empowers marginalized or underserved populations to share their experiences. When Wang (1999) developed photovoice, her primary goal was to give a voice to the voiceless. Wang and Burris (1997) assert that this is especially important for women, individuals experiencing social stigmas, and those not speaking the dominant language as they often have been overlooked in participatory research. Photovoice is a powerful approach to promote grassroots change, and I used the method in my study to explore what helps and hinders parents from getting their family to eat healthy and be physically active.

DESCRIPTION OF THE CURRENT STUDY

Past Research Using Photovoice

I discuss the main steps in the investigation and, first, would like to share with you some of the past research that has used photovoice as a data collection method. Photovoice has been used to elicit information about supportive or detrimental factors impacting health in a variety of populations: family planning for Midwestern Latino adults (Schwartz, Sable, Dannerbeck, & Campbell, 2007); family health of adults in Northern California (Wang & Pies, 2004); health concerns of college students in the Northeast (Goodhart et al., 2006); perceptions of health for preadolescent Latinas in the Midwest (Vaughn, Rojas-Guyler, & Howell, 2008); healthy eating for low-income homeless women in the Northeast (Valera, Gallin, Schuk, & Davis, 2009); perceptions of health for young adolescent mothers (Stevens, 2006); perceptions of health effects of environmental issues among indigenous community members in Western Canada (Castleden, Garvin, & Huu-ay-aht First Nation, 2008); and barriers and facilitators for people with spinal cord injury (Newman et al., 2009; Newman, 2010).

In the past 2 years, photovoice has also been used to explore immigrant residents' perceptions of neighborhood characteristics impacting health in Canada (Haque & Eng, 2011); barriers and facilitators in food purchasing and preparation among rural older adult women (Neill, Leipert, Garcia, & Kloseck, 2011); older adults' perceptions of psychosocial factors impacting physical activity (Mahmood et al., 2012), and the perspective of older adults on age-friendly communities in Canada (Novek, Morris-Oswald, & Menec, 2012). Photovoice has not been used with parents to share assets and barriers to healthy eating and physical activity, a gap that was filled by my study.

The primary aim of my study was to explore parental perceptions of assets and barriers to healthy eating and physical activity using photovoice as a data collection method. In the study, the three major goals were to have the participants produce images with their cameras, receive and attach meaning to the images, and contextualize the content of the images (Wang, 1999). Parents have an important role in helping their children to achieve a healthy lifestyle. Understanding parental perception on what helps and hinders healthy eating and physical activity is an important first step in being able to plan family-tailored interventions that meet the unique needs of the family unit.

Conceptual Issues

The literature was reviewed a priori for this study. I made this decision for several reasons. Because this was the first time I was using the photovoice data collection method, I needed to have a solid understanding of the method as well as of methodological issues. A thorough review of the literature was necessary to get a firm grasp of the philosophical underpinnings of the photovoice method. As a novice qualitative researcher, I needed detailed instructions on how to conduct a photovoice study. I was interested in having a basic knowledge of the types of populations that have been involved in photovoice studies and a general sense of the sample size needed.

After conducting the literature review, I was able to write a compelling argument for using photovoice as a methodology. I discovered that photovoice has not been used to document parental perceptions of assets and barriers to healthy eating and physical activity. My proposed study filled a gap in the literature, and I believed that it would be a valuable contribution to nursing science. My goal was to engage parents in a discussion about their family's health. The population of interest was parents who are patients of a nurse-run community clinic serving underinsured or uninsured individuals. I volunteer my time at the clinic as a registered nurse. I believed that by conducting my study at the clinic, I could give a voice to parents who have been marginalized as a result of language barriers, socioeconomic factors, and legal status issues. Because my goal is to build a family-tailored weight management intervention, I wanted to start at the grassroots level by giving the parents an opportunity to share what helps and hinders their family from eating healthy and being physically active.

As with most qualitative methods, a theoretical framework was not used to guide this study. The reason that a theoretical framework was not used a priori is that it may bias the researcher. If the researcher uses a theoretical framework to guide the study, the researcher may find him- or herself asking the participants guided questions or looking for specific themes during data analysis. Although this may be unintentional, it is best to let the theoretical framework emerge during data analysis.

METHODOLOGY

Design

As mentioned earlier, photography is a powerful tool for social change at the grassroots level. CBPR is about empowering individuals, families, communities, and populations to become involved with the change process. CBPR helps to open up a dialogue between the researcher and the participants about everyday life factors that impact health (Olshansky, 2008). The result of this dialogue is change at the community level.

CBPR is one type of qualitative methodology. The decision to use one qualitative design over another is driven by the research aims and/or research questions. My research aim was to explore parental perceptions of assets and barriers to healthy eating and physical activity; CBPR was the method of choice because it involved a critical dialogue about supportive and detrimental factors impacting health. Certainly I could have considered phenomenology to explore perceptions of factors from everyday life that impact healthy eating and physical activity. Although there is value in understanding an individual's lived experience, a criticism of using phenomenology has been that it may isolate an individual's experience without fully considering the sociocultural and historical context (Kirkham & Browne, 2006).

The photovoice data collection method allows the research participants to document through photography social, cultural, and economic factors impacting health. Photography is a powerful mechanism for an individual to express how he or she perceives the world. When someone is asked to take pictures, it gives the viewer a unique opportunity to see the world through that person's eyes. As the reseacher discusses the pictures with the participants, the researcher gets a chance to learn more about the context of the situation because of the visual aids. For example, the researcher can discuss healthy eating with a parent, but it is quite a different experience for the parent to present a photograph of the contents of their refrigerator as a way of demonstrating how he or she encourages healthy eating in the home.

Assumptions

As a researcher, it is important to address any assumptions before proceeding with the study. The primary assumption in this study was that people will tell the truth as they see it within their sociocultural context. Another assumption in this study involved the use of the word "healthy" and the phrase "physically active." I made the assumption that the meaning of the word "healthy" and the phrase "physically active" varied from person to person. A final assumption I made in this study was that socioeconomic factors were going to have a significant impact on a family's ability to eat a healthy diet and be physically active.

Sample

To conduct my study, I wrote grant proposals and successfully obtained a total of $4,000 worth of funding from two nursing organizations. Based on literature review and my readings about the photovoice methodology,

I proposed recruiting seven to ten research participants. I ultimately enrolled ten participants and had six complete the study. One reason for the small number of participants was the funding restriction. Because I initially planned to conduct focus groups as part of the research method, keeping the group between seven and ten participants would allow for a nice group discussion without becoming unwieldy. As a novice qualitative researcher, I wanted to make sure that I was able to manage the group dynamics, while encouraging all participants to become engaged in the discussion.

As mentioned previously, I recruited participants from a nurse-run community clinic near the university where I teach. My university supports the clinic administratively. Faculty members from the school of nursing and department of social work staff the clinic. The clinic provides primary health care and chronic disease management, serving individuals between the ages of 18 and 65 who meet certain income restrictions (at or below the poverty level). The patients who use the clinic's services are either uninsured or underinsured. Many of the patients served are homeless; the clinic works with a local religious organization that refers homeless persons from its shelter. About half of the patients from the clinic are originally from Mexico or Latin America, with a majority of these individuals speaking Spanish as their primary language.

For the past 2 years, I have volunteered my time at the clinic as a staff registered nurse. In this role, I triage and assess patients at their regularly scheduled visits and provide nursing care. This role has afforded me the opportunity to get to know most of our patients and the clinic staff. Gaining entrée into a community setting can be a challenge. Developing relationships within the community takes time and effort but is an essential first step in gaining entrée.

Prior to submitting my study proposal to the institutional review board (IRB) for approval, I ensured support from the clinic administrative director and staff. I met with the administrative director of the clinic to discuss the aims of my study and obtained support and permission to recruit my research participants. I discussed my research aims with the nurse practitioners at the clinic, the dietician, and the front office staff. The staff at the clinic was supportive of the project, and was instrumental in helping me recruit research participants. Developing relationships with the staff is an important step in the process. If you have buy-in from the staff, you are more likely to successfully recruit participants. If the staff trusts you, so will potential participants.

IRB Approval

When I had received permission to conduct my study, I prepared my application for IRB approval from my university. It is important to take the time to thoroughly read the IRB guidelines when preparing an application. Following my IRB's decision grid, I was able to submit my proposal under the exempt category, which means that the study poses minimal risk to the participants. In my application, I provided copies of my proposed consent form in both English and Spanish as many of the potential participants for the study were Spanish speaking. Because of the fact that photographs were going to be taken by the participants, I was careful to note how I would instruct the participants to take pictures. I also included English and Spanish versions of a photography consent form, in case my participants were going to take another individual's picture.

Because my study was in the exempt category, the review was conducted quickly, and I received approval for my study. After you receive approval for the study, it is important to keep the IRB informed of any changes necessary to make to the protocol. After I began to recruit my participants and collect data, I realized it was difficult to recruit participants for focus group sessions. I sent an addendum to the IRB requesting that I be allowed to conduct one-on-one interviews with participants as an alternative to focus groups. The IRB readily approved the change, and I made minor adjustments to the consent form. Sometimes modifications to the methodology are necessary; in this case it was better for some of my participants to be interviewed one-on-one as a result of their personal scheduling constraints.

IRB approval is only one mechanism of protecting research participants. Protecting participant privacy is important. Although I kept a master list of the participants, I was careful to separate signed research consent forms from the demographic questionnaires. While tape recording the focus groups or interview sessions, I did not use the participants' names. Some qualitative researchers give their participants pseudonyms, which are used throughout the study. All study materials including consent forms, demographic questionnaires, and tapes from the interviews should be kept in a locked drawer or somewhere else safe. It is also important to make sure that your computer is firewalled and password protected to ensure that participant data remain private. Finally, when publishing the results of the research, participants' names and identifying information are not used; findings are presented as aggregate data. It is, however, acceptable to use pseudonyms in publications as long as no one can identify the participants.

Setting

Recruitment, focus groups, and interviews all took place at the nurse-run community clinic. The clinic is located off a busy highway, adjacent to a local religious organization. Upon entering the clinic, patients check in with clinic staff at a window in a sizable waiting room. The clinic has four full-functioning exam rooms, two administrative offices, an office for mental health/social work staff, an office for the dietician, and a staff break room. There are two restrooms, one in the waiting room for the patients and one in the back for the staff. The building housing the clinic was opened in 2010; the space is modern and clean.

The focus groups were conducted in two spaces: the waiting room (after business hours) and the mental health/social work office. The decision was made to use the waiting room for the first focus group meeting because of the size of the room and the ample number of chairs. During a subsequent focus group, I made the decision to use the mental health/social work office because the group was small in size.

The initial two focus groups were conducted in the evening after normal clinic business hours. The evening hours were selected so that the time did not conflict with parents needing to pick up children from school or day care. Parents were encouraged to bring their children. I provided babysitting services so that I could have the parents' full attention during the focus group sessions.

I hired high school- and college-aged students to babysit. The babysitters had to apply for a child care position at the university. As part of the application process, a background check was completed. Babysitters had to produce evidence of cardiopulmonary resuscitation (CPR) certification that was current (within the last 2 years). Background checks and CPR certification requirements ensured that the babysitters were qualified to provide child care services, protecting both the children and the parents. If the parents opted to take advantage of the babysitting services, they were required to sign a consent form for babysitting, releasing the university from liability. The consent form for babysitting was drafted by the university's legal department. The dietician's office was used for babysitting. The table was covered with a tablecloth and I provided crayons, coloring books, and games.

Because I opted to conduct the focus group meetings in the early evening, I provided food for the participants and their children. I brought a light dinner meal including sandwiches, crackers, fruit, vegetables, juice, and water. The clinic only has one small staff refrigerator. I had to plan on bringing coolers and ice to keep the food cold. Another challenge with providing food is the amount. During the first two focus groups, I had a great deal of food left over, which I decided to send home with the participants.

Data Collection

I now describe in detail the steps of the data collection process. Wang's (1999) steps of the photovoice method were used. After receiving IRB approval, the first step was to recruit participants from the community health clinic. With the help of the clinic staff, I approached regularly scheduled patients who had children between the ages of 2 and 19 years to ascertain their interest in participating in the study. Spanish-speaking interpreters hired by the clinic assisted me with the communication. The decision was made to use Spanish-speaking interpreters hired by the clinic because the patients are familiar with the interpreters. Participants who expressed interest in participating in the study were given a copy of the consent form to read. After they read the consent form, potential participants had an opportunity to ask questions before signing the form. Copies of the consent form was given to the participants for their reference.

After ten participants were recruited, the second step was to schedule an initial session to introduce the participants to the photovoice method including how to use the cameras, how to take meaningful photographs, and ethical concerns with photography in the community (e.g., not taking someone's picture without their permission). Each participant was assigned a participant number (e.g., 01). I kept a master list of participant names and numbers. Participants were called a week before the initial session and the day before the initial session to remind them of the date, time, and location of the session. Despite reminder calls, only four of the ten originally scheduled participants showed up for the initial session.

During the initial orientation session, demographic information, including age, gender, marital status, employment status, income level, number of children, and children's height and weight to determine their children's BMI, was collected from each participant. Demographic information was collected to describe the sample. After the participants filled out the demographic questionnaire, I introduced the interpreter and notified the participants that I would be recording the session. A digital voice recorder was set up in the center of the room. I discussed the importance of having only one person speak at a time. After turning on the digital recorder, each participant was given a binder, one disposable camera, and a notebook to record notes or insights while taking the pictures. The binder contained instructions for taking photographs and photography consent forms in English and Spanish. The photography consent forms were important to include in case the participant took photographs of people. As a group, we discussed the instructions on how to take meaningful photographs (e.g., not covering the lens with the finger, not needing to center all of the objects of interest), and how to use the cameras. Ethical photography was also discussed.

As part of the initial session, the participants and I posed themes related to the topic of healthy/unhealthy eating and physical activity in their homes and communities. As a group, we discussed ideas for photographs. Participant questions were answered during this time. The participants were instructed to take six to seven pictures on each subtheme including (a) persons, places, and things that helped their family eat healthy; (b) persons, places, and things that prevented their family from eating healthy; (c) persons, places, or things that helped their family be physically active; and (d) persons, places, or things that prevented their family from being physically active. Throughout the initial discussion, I took copious notes. The participants were given an approximate time period of 1 month to take the photographs and return the cameras to the clinic in an envelope provided in their binder.

As part of this process, I quickly realized that, despite interest in the study and reminder phone calls, scheduling constraints for focus groups were an issue. I amended my IRB application to include individual interviews as an additional method of recruiting and collecting data. The final six participants were recruited individually. The instruction sessions were given one-on-one and audio recorded.

The third step involved sending the disposable cameras for processing. Once the participants dropped off the cameras at the clinic, I took the disposable cameras for processing. The participant's ID number was used as an identifier. For each participant I had two sets of pictures made. A copy of their pictures was put on a disc. Once I had the developed photographs I scheduled a second focus group (for the first four participants) or individual interviews.

The fourth step involved meeting with participants for the second focus group or interview. Each participant selected three to five photographs to share with the group (or with me) on a combination of any, or all, of the subthemes. The session was recorded with the digital voice recorder, and I took copious notes throughout. To contextualize and tell stories about the pictures, the acronym "SHOWeD" (Wang & Burris, 1997) was used to guide the participants as they shared each of their photographs: (a) What do you See here? (b) What is really Happening here? (c) How does this relate to Our lives? (d) Why does this situation, concern, or strength exist? and (e) What can we do about it?

After the participants had an opportunity to discuss each of their pictures, I opened up a time to share general comments about what helps and hinders their families from eating healthy and being physically active. At the conclusion of the dialogue, I summarized general themes that were shared by the group or an individual as a way of member checking and maintaining rigor in the study. Member checking is an important step in the process; it is essential that the participants understand that their voices are heard. Member checking gives the participants the opportunity to address concerns or correct information that they felt was not an accurate representation of what was shared.

An integral part of the data collection process is reflective journaling. As I began the study, I kept a journal of my thoughts about the study procedures including aspects of the study that I felt were successful and aspects of the study that were challenging. In the journal, I addressed what I might do differently the next time. In addition to helping establish an audit trail, journaling provides an opportunity to document the researcher's thoughts, feelings, and impressions. In the journaling process the researcher has the opportunity to reflect on preconceived notions and potential biases that may interfere with data collection or data analysis.

Timeline

Prior to beginning a research investigation, it is important to establish a timeline for the completion of the project. Proposing a timeline will help the researcher to stay on track and finish the project in a timely fashion. When a researcher obtains funding for research projects, as I did for this study, there will be budgetary time constraints. If a researcher is employed by a university, research funds are awarded to the university rather than to the individual. If the university has an office of research, funding received will be managed through the office of research. The awarded grant is likely to have stipulations about when and how research money is to be spent. By writing a realistic timeline, the researcher is able to ensure that the project is completed within the timeframe outlined by the research grant guidelines.

Table 10.1 is an example of the timeline used for this study. In writing a timeline for this study, I gave myself 1 year to complete the project. The 1-year timeline also met the funding requirements.

As part of the research process, it is realistic to expect that there will be challenges faced in participant recruitment and retention. Participant attrition was a particular challenge in this study because the participants were asked to take photographs, return their cameras, and attend a follow-up focus group or interview session. I initially recruited ten participants, with six completing the project. I attempted to reduce attrition by making follow-up phone calls to the participants and by arranging one-on-one interviews during or after regularly scheduled clinic appointments. I made every effort to work around my participants' schedules.

Table 10.1 *Timeline for Study*

Specific Activities or Steps	Month of Activity or Step (Year–Year)											
	Jul	Aug	Sept	Oct	Nov	Dec	Jan	Feb	Mar	Apr	May	June
Obtain IRB approval	X											
Sample selection	X	X										
First focus group			X									
Participants take pictures				X								
Second focus group					X							
Data transcription						X	X					
Data analysis and interpretation								X	X	X		
Community sharing											X	
Dissemination of findings											X	X→

Data Analysis

The study was designed to amass rich data from each participant's unique perspective about familial assets and barriers to healthy eating and physical activity. Ethnocentric bias is a concern in conducting qualitative research. To reduce ethnocentric bias in the research, I bracketed my preconceived notions or assumptions to prevent misinterpretation of the data. Bracketing is the process of being open to analyzing the data by taking steps to acknowledge one's beliefs, judgments, and preconceived notions (Speziale & Carpenter, 2002).

As part of the reflective journaling process I discussed my preconceived notions and assumptions through the process of narrative self-disclosure. I wrote down my beliefs about possible barriers and facilitators to healthy eating and physical activity (e.g., economic factors, the fact that there may be cultural differences). After I wrote down my beliefs and assumptions, I reflected on how my personal values would impact the study. I devised a plan to strictly follow the "SHOWeD" script and attempted not to ask leading questions during the focus groups or interviews. It was important to let the participants tell their stories.

Data were analyzed using Diekelman, Allen, and Tanner's (1989) procedural steps. Because I was a novice qualitative researcher, I enlisted the help of an experienced qualitative researcher who assisted me with data collection and data analysis. The experienced qualitative researcher was my co-investigator in this study.

The first step was to have the audio-recorded focus group sessions and interviews transcribed by a bilingual transcriptionist. Any transcripts with Spanish were translated into English by the transcriptionist. The transcripts were retranslated back to Spanish to ensure accuracy.

Second, the interview transcripts and field notes were read in their entirety to gain an overall impression. The transcripts and photographs were imported into the software program NVivo 9. In NVivo, data are analyzed by identifying nodes or themes within the transcripts. The software helps you to organize the nodes or themes.

Third, my coinvestigator and I summarized the key findings and searched for general themes. The photographs were included in the analysis for reference.

Fourth, we reviewed the transcripts and NVivo output together. Common nodes/themes were identified.

Fifth, we identified emerging patterns among the previously coded nodes/themes. Each of the finally identified themes had one or two corresponding photographs selected to highlight the theme.

The last step involved making a final interpretation of the data and making plans for the dissemination of the data.

Dissemination

As part of the CBPR process the participants can be engaged in a review of the results. A plan is made to disseminate the results to advisory board members at the community clinic. Sharing can provide the impetus to start the process of change and to plan for a family-tailored weight management intervention. The meeting will give the participants an opportunity to share what they have learned and dialogue about changes they will make to improve the health of their families. The discussion time will also give the group a chance to dialogue about specific ideas and plan for a family-tailored weight management intervention, addressing areas of need identified during the study.

CONCLUSION

In conclusion, CBPR can be an effective method to empower individuals, families, communities, and populations to make meaningful health-related changes. As you have learned, a CBPR approach, employing the photovoice data collection method, has been used to explore facilitators and barriers to health among a variety of populations in diverse settings. Giving a voice to the voiceless is a powerful way of opening up a dialogue, which can lead to change at the community level.

REFERENCES

Castleden, H., Garvin, T., & Huu-ay-aht First Nation. (2008). Modifying Photovoice for community-based participatory Indigenous research. *Social Science & Medicine, 66,* 1393–1405. doi:10.1016/j.socscimed.2007.11.030

Diekelman, N. L., Allen, D., & Tanner, C. (1989). *The NLN criteria for appraisal of baccalaureate programs: Critical hermeneutic analysis.* New York, NY: National League for Nursing.

Freire, P. (1970). *Pedagogy of the oppressed.* New York, NY: Continuum International Publishing Group, Inc.

Golan, M., & Crow, S. (2004). Parents are key players in the prevention and treatment of weight-related problems. *Nutrition Reviews, 82,* 39–50.

Goodhart, F. W., Hsu, J., Baek, J. H., Coleman, A. L., Maresca, F. M., & Miller, M. B. (2006). A view through a different lens: Photovoice as a tool for student advocacy. *Journal of American College Health, 55*, 53–56.

Haque, N., & Eng, B. (2011). Tackling inequity through a Photovoice project on the social determinants of health: Translating Photovoice evidence to community action. *Global Health Promotion, 18*, 16–19. doi:10.1177/1757975910393165

Kirkham, S. R., & Browne, A. J. (2006). Towards a critical theoretical interpretation of social justice discourses in nursing. *Advances in Nursing Science, 29*, 324–329.

Mahmood, A., Chaudhury, H., Michael, Y. L., Campo, M., Hay, K., & Sarte, A. (2012). A Photovoice documentation of the role of neighborhood physical and social environments in older adults' physical activity in two metropolitan areas in North America. *Social Science & Medicine, 74*, 1180–1992. doi:10.1016/j.socscimed.2011.12.039

Neill, C., Leipert, B. D., Garcia, A. C., & Kloseck, M. (2011). Using Photovoice methodology to investigate facilitators and barriers to food acquisition and preparation in rural older women. *Journal of Nutrition in Gerontology and Geriatrics, 30*, 225–247. doi:10.1080/21551197.2011.591268

Newman, S. D. (2010). Evidence-based advocacy: Using Photovoice to identify barriers and facilitators to community participation after spinal cord injury. *Rehabilitation Nursing, 35*(2), 47–59.

Newman, S., Maurer, D., Jackson, A., Saxon, M., Jones, R., & Reese, G. (2009). Gathering the evidence: Photovoice as a tool for disability advocacy. *Progress in Community Health Partnerships: Research, Education, and Action, 3*(2), 139–144.

Novek, S., Morris-Oswald, T., & Menec, V. (2012). Using Photovoice with older adults: Some methodologic strengths and issues. *Ageing and Society, 32*, 451–470.

Ogden, C. L., Carroll, M. D., Curtin, L. R., Lamb, M. M., & Flegal, K. M. (2010). Prevalence of high body mass index in US children and adolescents, 2007–2008. *The Journal of the American Medical Association, 303*, 242–249.

Olshansky, E. (2008). The use of community based participatory research to understand and work with vulnerable populations. In M. de Chesnay & B. A. Anderson, (Eds.) *Caring for the vulnerable: Perspectives in nursing theory, practice, and research* (2nd ed.). Sudbury, MA: Jones and Bartlett Publishers.

Schwartz, L., Sable, M., Dannerbeck, A., & Campbell, J. (2007). Using Photovoice to improve family planning for immigrant Hispanics. *Journal for Health Care of the Poor and Underserved, 18*, 757–766.

Speziale, H. J., & Carpenter, D. R. (2002). *Qualitative research in nursing: Advancing the humanistic imperative* (3rd ed.). Philadelphia, PA: Lippincott Williams & Wilkins.

Stevens, C. A. (2006). Being healthy: Voices of adolescent women who are parenting. *Journal for Specialists in Pediatric Nursing, 11*, 28–40.

Valera, P., Gallin, J., Schuk, D., & Davis, N. (2009). "Trying to eat healthy": A Photovoice study about women's access to healthy food in New York City. *Affilia: Journal of Women and Social Work, 24*, 300–314.

Vaughn, L., Rojas-Guyler, L., & Howell, B. (2008). "Picturing" health: A Photovoice pilot of Latina girls' perceptions of health. *Family and Community Health, 31*, 305–316. doi:10.1097/01.FCH.0000336093.39066.e9

Wang, C. C. (1999). Photovoice: A participatory action research strategy applied to women's health. *Journal of Women's Health, 8,* 185–192.

Wang, C., & Burris, M. (1997). Photovoice: Concept, methodology, and use for participatory needs assessment. *Health Education & Behavior, 24,* 369–378.

Wang, C. C., & Pies, C. M. (2004). Family, maternal, and child health through Photovoice. *Maternal and Child Health Journal, 8,* 95–102.

Weiler, K. (1988). *Women teaching for change: Gender, class, and power.* South Hadley, MA: Bergin and Garvey.

LIST OF JOURNALS THAT PUBLISH QUALITATIVE RESEARCH

Mary de Chesnay

Conducting excellent research and not publishing the results negates the study and prohibits anyone from learning from the work. Therefore, it is critical that qualitative researchers disseminate their work widely, and the best way to do so is through publication in refereed journals. The peer review process, although seemingly brutal at times, is designed to improve knowledge by enhancing the quality of literature in a discipline. Fortunately, the publishing climate has evolved to the point where qualitative research is valued by editors and readers alike, and many journals now seek out, or even specialize in publishing, qualitative research.

The following table was compiled partially from the synopsis of previous work identifying qualitative journals by the St. Louis University Qualitative Research Committee (2013), with a multidisciplinary faculty, who are proponents of qualitative research. Many of these journals would be considered multidisciplinary, though marketed to nurses. All are peer reviewed. Other journals were identified by the author of this series and by McKibbon and Gadd (2004) in their quantitative analysis of qualitative research. It is not meant to be exhaustive, and we would welcome any suggestions for inclusion.

An additional resource is the nursing literature mapping project conducted by Sherwill-Navarro and Allen (Allen, Jacobs, & Levy, 2006). The 217 journals were listed as a resource for libraries to accrue relevant journals, and many of them publish qualitative research. Readers are encouraged to view the websites for specific journals that might be interested in publishing their studies. Readers are also encouraged to look outside the traditional nursing journals, especially if their topics more closely match the journal mission of related disciplines.

NURSING JOURNALS

Journal	Website
Advances in Nursing Science	www.journals.lww.com/advancesinnursingscience/pages/default.aspx
Africa Journal of Nursing and Midwifery	www.journals.co.za/ej/ejour_ajnm.html
Annual Review of Nursing Research	www.springerpub.com/product/07396686#.UeaXbjvvv6U
British Journal of Nursing	www.britishjournalofnursing.com
Canadian Journal of Nursing Research	www.cjnr.mcgill.ca
Hispanic Health Care International	www.springerpub.com/product/15404153#.UeaX7jvvv6U
Holistic Nursing Practice	www.journals.lww.com/hnpjournal/pages/default.aspx
International Journal of Mental Health Nursing	www.onlinelibrary.wiley.com/journal/10.1111/(ISSN)1447-0349
International Journal of Nursing Practice	www.onlinelibrary.wiley.com/journal/10.1111/(ISSN)1440-172X
International Journal of Nursing Studies	www.journals.elsevier.com/international-journal-of-nursing-studies
Journal of Advanced Nursing	www.onlinelibrary.wiley.com/journal/10.1111/(ISSN)1365-2648
Journal of Clinical Nursing	www.onlinelibrary.wiley.com/journal/10.1111/(ISSN)1365-2702
Journal of Family Nursing	www.jfn.sagepub.com
Journal of Nursing Education	www.healio.com/journals/JNE
Journal of Nursing Scholarship	www.onlinelibrary.wiley.com/journal/10.1111/(ISSN)1547-5069
Nurse Researcher	www.nurseresearcher.rcnpublishing.co.uk
Nursing History Review	www.aahn.org/nhr.html
Nursing Inquiry	www.onlinelibrary.wiley.com/journal/10.1111/(ISSN)1440-1800
Nursing Research	www.ninr.nih.gov
Nursing Science Quarterly	www.nsq.sagepub.com
Online Brazilian Journal of Nursing	www.objnursing.uff.br/index.php/nursing

(continued)

Journal	Website
The Online Journal of Cultural Competence in Nursing and Healthcare	www.ojccnh.org
Public Health Nursing	www.onlinelibrary.wiley.com/journal/10.1111/(ISSN)1525-1446
Qualitative Health Research	www.qhr.sagepub.com
Qualitative Research in Nursing and Healthcare	www.wiley.com/WileyCDA/WileyTitle/product Cd-1405161221.html
Research and Theory for Nursing Practice	www.springerpub.com/product/15416577#.Ueab lTvvv6U
Scandinavian Journal of Caring Sciences	www.onlinelibrary.wiley.com/journal/10.1111/(ISSN)1471-6712
Western Journal of Nursing Research	http://wjn.sagepub.com

REFERENCES

Allen, M., Jacobs, S. K., & Levy, J. R. (2006). Mapping the literature of nursing: 1996–2000. *Journal of the Medical Library Association, 94*(2), 206–220. Retrieved from http://nahrs.mlanet.org/home/images/activity/nahrs2012selectedlist nursing.pdf

McKibbon, K., & Gadd, C. (2004). A quantitative analysis of qualitative studies in clinical journals for the publishing year 2000. *BMC Med Inform Decision Making, 4*, 11. Retrieved from http://www.ncbi.nlm.nih.gov/pmc/articles/PMC503397

St. Louis University Qualitative Research Committee. Retrieved July 14, 2013, from http://www.slu.edu/organizations/qrc/QRjournals.html

ESSENTIAL ELEMENTS FOR A QUALITATIVE PROPOSAL

Tommie Nelms

1. Introduction: Aim of the study
   a. Phenomenon of interest and focus of inquiry
   b. Justification for studying the phenomenon (how big an issue/problem?)
   c. Phenomenon discussed within a specific context (lived experience, culture, human response)
   d. Theoretical framework(s)
   e. Assumptions, biases, experiences, intuitions, and perceptions related to the belief that inquiry into a phenomenon is important (researcher's relationship to the topic)
   f. Qualitative methodology chosen, with rationale
   g. Significance to nursing (How will the new knowledge gained benefit patients, nursing practice, nurses, society, etc.?)
   Note: The focus of interest/inquiry and statement of purpose of the study should appear at the top of page 3 of the proposal
2. Literature review: What is known about the topic? How has it been studied in the past?
   Include background of the theoretical framework and how it has been used in the past.
3. Methodology
   a. Introduction of methodology (philosophical underpinnings of the method)
   b. Rationale for choosing the methodology
   c. Background of methodology
   d. Outcome of methodology
   e. Methods: general sources, and steps and procedures
   f. Translation of concepts and terms

4. Methods
    a. Aim
    b. Participants
    c. Setting
    d. Gaining access, and recruitment of participants
    e. General steps in conduct of study (data gathering tool(s), procedures, etc.)
    f. Human subjects' considerations
    g. Expected timetable
    h. Framework for rigor, and specific strategies to ensure rigor
    i. Plans and procedures for data analysis

WRITING QUALITATIVE RESEARCH PROPOSALS

Joan L. Bottorff

PURPOSE OF A RESEARCH PROPOSAL

- Communicates research plan to others (e.g., funding agencies)
- Serves as a detailed plan of action
- Serves as a contract between investigator and funding bodies when proposal is approved

QUALITATIVE RESEARCH: BASIC ASSUMPTIONS

- Reality is complex, constructed, and, ultimately, subjective.
- Research is an interpretative process.
- Knowledge is best achieved by conducting research in the natural setting.

QUALITATIVE RESEARCH

- Qualitative research is unstructured.
- Qualitative designs are "emergent" rather than fixed.
- The results of qualitative research are unpredictable (Morse, 1994).

KINDS OF QUALITATIVE RESEARCH

- Grounded theory
- Ethnography (critical ethnography, institutional ethnography, ethno-methodology, ethnoscience, etc.)
- Phenomenology
- Narrative inquiry
- Others

CHALLENGES FOR QUALITATIVE RESEARCHERS

- Developing a solid, convincing argument that the study contributes to theory, research, practice, and/or policy (the "so what?" question)
- Planning a study that is systematic, manageable, and flexible (to reassure skeptics):
  - Justification of the selected qualitative method
  - Explicit details about design and methods, without limiting the project's evolution
  - Attention to criteria for the overall soundness or rigor of the project

QUESTIONS A PROPOSAL MUST ANSWER

- Why should anyone be interested in my research?
- Is the research design credible, achievable, and carefully explained?
- Is the researcher capable of conducting the research? (Marshall & Rossman, 1999)

TIPS TO ANSWER THESE QUESTIONS

- Be practical (practical problems cannot be easily brushed off)
- Be persuasive ("sell" your proposal)
- Make broad links (hint at the wider context)
- Aim for crystal clarity (avoid jargon, assume nothing, explain everything) (Silverman, 2000)

SECTIONS OF A TYPICAL QUALITATIVE PROPOSAL

- Introduction
  - Introduction of topic and its significance
  - Statement of purpose, research questions/objectives
- Review of literature
  - Related literature and theoretical traditions
- Design and methods
  - Overall approach and rationale
  - Sampling, data gathering methods, data analysis
  - Trustworthiness (soundness of the research)
  - Ethical considerations
- Dissemination and knowledge translation
  - Timeline
  - Budget
  - Appendices

INTRODUCING THE STUDY—FIRST PARA

- Goal: Capture interest in the study
  - Focus on the importance of the study (Why bother with the question?)
  - Be clear and concise (details will follow)
  - Provide a synopsis of the primary target of the study
  - Present persuasive logic backed up with factual evidence

THE PROBLEM/RESEARCH QUESTION

- The problem can be broad, but it must be specific enough to convince others that it is worth focusing on.
- Research questions must be clearly delineated.
- The research questions must sometimes be delineated with sub-questions.
- The scope of the research question(s) needs to be manageable within the time frame and context of the study.

PURPOSE OF THE QUALITATIVE STUDY

- Discovery?
- Description?
- Conceptualization (theory building)?
- Sensitization?
- Emancipation?
- Other?

LITERATURE REVIEW

- The literature review should be selective and persuasive, building a case for what is known or believed, what is missing, and how the study fits in.
- The literature is used to demonstrate openness to the complexity of the phenomenon, rather than funneling toward an a priori conceptualization.

METHODS—CHALLENGES HERE

- Quantitative designs are often more familiar to reviewers.
- Qualitative researchers have a different language.

METHODS SECTION

- Orientation to the method:
  - Description of the particular method that will be used and its creators/interpreters
  - Rationale for qualitative research generally and for the specific method to be used

QUALITATIVE STUDIES ARE VALUABLE FOR RESEARCH

- It delves deeply into complexities and processes.
- It focuses on little-known phenomena or innovative systems.

- It explores informal and unstructured processes in organizations.
- It seeks to explore where and why policy and local knowledge and practice are at odds.
- It is based on real, as opposed to stated, organizational goals.
- It cannot be done experimentally for practical or ethical reasons.
- It requires identification of relevant variables (Marshall & Rossman, 1999).

SAMPLE

- Purposive or theoretical sampling
  - The purpose of the sampling
  - Characteristics of potential types of persons, events, or processes to be sampled
  - Methods of making decisions about sampling
- Sample size
  - Estimates provided based on previous experience, pilot work, etc.
- Access and recruitment

DATA COLLECTION AND ANALYSIS

- Types: Individual interviews, participant observation, focus groups, personal and public documents, Internet-based data, videos, and so on, all of which vary with different traditions.
- Analysis methods vary depending on the qualitative approach.
- Add DETAILS and MORE DETAILS about how data will be gathered and processed (procedures should be made public).

QUESTIONS FOR DATA MANAGEMENT AND ANALYSIS

- How will data be kept organized and retrievable?
- How will data be "broken up" to see something new?
- How will the researchers engage in reflexivity (e.g., be self-analytical)?
- How will the reader be convinced that the researcher is sufficiently knowledgeable about qualitative analysis and has the necessary skills?

TRUSTWORTHINESS (SOUNDNESS OF THE RESEARCH)

- Should be reflected throughout the proposal
- Should be addressed specifically, with the relevant criteria for the qualitative approach used
- Should provide examples of the strategies used:
  - Triangulation
  - Prolonged contact with informants, including continuous validation of data
  - Continuous checking for representativeness of data and fit between coding categories and data
  - Use of expert consultants

EXAMPLES OF STRATEGIES FOR LIMITING BIAS IN INTERPRETATIONS

- Planning to search for negative cases
- Describing how analysis will include a purposeful examination of alternative explanations
- Using members of the research team to critically question the analysis
- Planning to conduct an audit of data collection and analytic strategies

OTHER COMPONENTS

- Ethical considerations
  - Consent forms
  - Dealing with sensitive issues
- Dissemination and knowledge translation
- Timeline
- Budget justification

LAST BITS OF ADVICE

- Seek assistance and pre-review from others with experience in grant writing (plan time for rewriting).
- Highlight match between your proposal and purpose of competition.
- Follow the rules of the competition.
- Write for a multidisciplinary audience.

REFERENCES

Marshall, C., & Rossman, G. B. (1999). *Designing qualitative research*. Thousand Oaks, CA: Sage.

Morse, J. M. (1994). Designing funded qualitative research. In N. Denzin & Y. Lincoln (Eds.), *Handbook of qualitative research* (pp. 220–235). Thousand Oaks, CA: Sage.

Silverman, D. (2000). *Doing qualitative research*. Thousand Oaks, CA: Sage.

OUTLINE FOR A RESEARCH PROPOSAL

Mary de Chesnay

The following guidelines are meant as a general set of suggestions that supplement the instructions for the student's program. In all cases where there is conflicting advice, the student should be guided by the dissertation chair's instructions. The outlined plan includes five chapters: the first three constitute the proposal and the remaining two the results and conclusions, but the number may vary depending on the nature of the topic or the style of the committee chair (e.g., I do not favor repeating the research questions at the beginning of every chapter, but some faculty do. I like to use this outline but some faculty prefer a different order. Some studies lend themselves to four instead of five chapters.).

Chapter I: Overview of the Study (or Preview of Coming Attractions) is a few pages that tell the reader:

- What he or she is going to investigate (purpose or statement of the problem and research questions or hypotheses).
- What theoretical support the idea has (conceptual framework or theoretical support). In qualitative research, this section may include only a rationale for conducting the study, with the conceptual framework or typology emerging from the data.
- What assumptions underlie the problem.
- What definitions of terms are important to state (typically, these definitions in quantitative research are called *operational definitions* because they describe how one will know the item when one sees it. An operational definition usually starts with the phrase: "a score of ... or above on the [name of instrument]"). One may also want to include a conceptual definition, which is the usual meaning of the concept of interest or a definition according to a specific author. In contrast, qualitative research usually does not include measurements, so operational definitions are not appropriate, but conceptual definitions may be important to state.

- What limitations to the design are expected (not delimitations, which are intentional decisions about how to narrow the scope of one's population or focus).
- What the importance of the study (significance) is to the discipline.

Chapter II: The Review of Research Literature (or Why You Are Not Reinventing the Wheel)

For Quantitative Research:
Organize this chapter according to the concepts in the conceptual framework in Chapter I and describe the literature review thoroughly first, followed by the state of the art of the literature and how the study fills the gaps in the existing literature. Do not include non research literature in this section—place it in Chapter I as introductory material if the citation is necessary to the description.

- Concept 1: a brief description of each study reviewed that supports concept 1 with appropriate transitional statements between paragraphs
- Concept 2: a brief description of each study reviewed that supports concept 2 with appropriate transitional statements between paragraphs
- Concept 3: a brief description of each study reviewed that supports concept 3 with appropriate transitional statements between paragraphs
- And so on, for as many concepts as there are in the conceptual framework (I advise limiting the number of concepts for a master's degree thesis owing to time and cost constraints)
- Areas of agreement in the literature—a paragraph, or two, that summarizes the main points on which authors agree
- Areas of disagreement—where the main issues on which authors disagree are summarized
- State of the art on the topic—a few paragraphs in which the areas where the literature is strong and where the gaps are, are clearly articulated
- A brief statement of how the study fills the gaps or why the study needs to be conducted to replicate what someone else has done

For Qualitative Research:
The literature review is usually conducted after the results are analyzed and the emergent concepts are known. The literature may then be placed in Chapter II of the proposal as shown earlier or incorporated into the results and discussion.

Chapter III: Methodology (or Exactly What You Are Going to Do Anyway)

- Design (name the design—e.g., ethnographic, experimental, survey, cross-sectional, phenomenological, grounded theory, etc.).
- Sample—describe the number of people who will serve as the sample and the sampling method: Where and how will the sample be recruited? Provide the rationale for sample selection and methods. Include the institutional review board (IRB) statement and say how the rights of subjects (Ss) will be protected, including how informed consent will be obtained and the data coded and stored.
- Setting—where will data collection take place? In quantitative research, this might be a laboratory or, if a questionnaire, a home. If qualitative, there are special considerations of privacy and comfortable surroundings for the interviews.
- Instruments and data analysis—how will the variables of interest be measured and how will sense be made of the data, if quantitative, and if qualitative, how will the data be coded and interpreted—that is, for both, this involves how the data will be analyzed.
- Validity and reliability—how will it be known if the data are good (in qualitative research, these terms are "accuracy" and "replicability").
- Procedures for data collection and analysis: a 1-2-3 step-by-step plan for what will be done.
- Timeline—a chart that lists the plan month by month—use Month 1, 2, 3 instead of January, February, March.

The above three-chapter plan constitutes an acceptable proposal for a research project. The following is an outline for the final two chapters.

Chapter IV: Results (What I Discovered)

- Some researchers like to describe the sample in this section as a way to lead off talking about the findings.
- In the order of each hypothesis or research question, describe the data that addressed that question. Use raw data only; do not conclude anything about the data and make no interpretations.

Chapter V: Discussion (or How I Can Make Sense of All This)

- Conclusions—a concise statement of the answer to each research question or hypothesis. Some people like to interpret here—that is, to say how confident they can be about each conclusion.

- Implications—how each conclusion can be used to help address the needs of vulnerable populations or nursing practice, education, or administration.
- Recommendations for further research—that is, what will be done for an encore?

INDEX